Infection Prevention and Control

PERCEPTIONS AND PERSPECTIVES

Edited by

PAUL ELLIOTT
RGN, BSc, MA, PGCEA, FHEA
Senior Lecturer in Adult Nursing and Infection Control
School of Nursing, Faculty of Health and Wellbeing
Canterbury Christ Church University, Kent

JULIE STORR
BN (Hons), RGN, MBA
Director, S3 Global
Consultant, World Health Organization
Past President, Infection Prevention Society
S3 Global, London

ANNETTE JEANES
RGN, MSc, Dip N, Dip IC
Director of Infection Prevention and Control
Consultant Nurse, Department of Infection Control
University College London Hospitals NHS Foundation Trust

Forewords by
PROFESSOR BARRY COOKSON
Honorary Professor
Epidemiology & Population Health Faculty
London School of Hygiene and Tropical Medicine

PROFESSOR BENEDETTA ALLEGRANZI
Lead, Clean Care is Safer Care and Infection Control Programme
Service Delivery and Safety Department
World Health Organization
Geneva

ADJ PROFESSOR MARILYN CRUICKSHANK
Director, National Healthcare Associated Infection Program
Australian Commission on Safety and Quality in Health Care

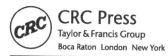

CRC Press
Taylor & Francis Group
Boca Raton London New York

CRC Press is an imprint of the
Taylor & Francis Group, an **informa** business

CRC Press
Taylor & Francis Group
6000 Broken Sound Parkway NW, Suite 300
Boca Raton, FL 33487-2742

© 2016 Paul Elliott, Julie Storr and Annette Jeanes
CRC Press is an imprint of Taylor & Francis Group, an Informa business

No claim to original U.S. Government works

Printed on acid-free paper
Version Date: 20150710

International Standard Book Number-13: 978-184619-989-9

Visit the Taylor & Francis Web site at
http://www.taylorandfrancis.com

and the CRC Press Web site at
http://www.crcpress.com

Contents

Foreword by Barry Cookson

Healthcare-associated infection and the related issues of antimicrobial resistance were considered for many years to be Cinderellas of medicine and public health. When I was first employed by the Public Health Laboratory Service in 1990 they did not even appear in that organisation's first business plan. Both are now recognised as major global threats to patient safety and national economies.

An interesting question to ask of any healthcare worker is which books changed their lives. For me it was Balint's *The Doctor, His Patient and the Illness*[1] and for some of my nursing colleagues, it was Walsh and Ford's *Nursing Rituals, Research and Rational Actions*.[2] Both are, of course, many years out of date, but still worth reading today, emphasising as they do the sociological aspects of the art of medicine.

This book, I would predict, will serve in a similar role to countless infection prevention and control practitioners. The editors, three experienced healthcare educators, have led by example in writing, and gathering together, a very talented and expert multi-disciplinary group of fellow authors to produce a provocative and highly stimulating book. Indeed, it should be essential reading for infection control-related courses, and the exercises that are included will serve well for practitioners' continuing professional development for years to come. The references are well-chosen, many of which would otherwise be hard to find. Readers will best benefit if they have a good background knowledge of the evidence base for infection prevention and control and related issues of antimicrobial stewardship.

If used in these ways, the book will make a major contribution in helping to develop infection prevention and control specialists with the competencies to work within a multi-disciplinary orchestra of healthcare workers capable of preventing and controlling the multi-faceted problems posed by healthcare-associated infection and antimicrobial resistance. This book also points out that this orchestra must be aware that their audience: the patients, their families and representatives, have a key role to play in informing how best to deliver healthcare and infection prevention and control services. We will then be equipped to address proactively and reactively as required, the 'highly complex combination of physical, psychological and social processes' described in this admirable book.

Professor Barry Cookson
Honorary Professor
Epidemiology & Population Health Faculty
London School of Hygiene and Tropical Medicine
July 2015

REFERENCES

1 Balint M. *The Doctor, His Patient and the Illness.* 2nd ed. London: Pitman; 1964. Millennium Edition. Edinburgh: Churchill Livingstone; 2000.
2 Walsh M, Ford P. *Nursing Rituals, Research and Rational Actions.* Oxford: Heinemann Nursing; 1989.

Foreword by Benedetta Allegranzi

Infection prevention and control (IPC) is vital in saving lives. As the lead for the IPC Programme *Clean Care is Safer Care* at WHO, I am committed to supporting those working every day to play a critical role in patient and health worker safety through IPC improvements. The evidence tells us that multifaceted approaches will prevent the avoidable infections that occur across the world every year. But from understanding determinants and risk factors to measuring outcomes, IPC is a complex science and gaps remain in the evidence base, particularly through good-quality research. While we need to accelerate the research that will allow more lives to be saved in every country, this should not paralyse us in considering and challenging current realities. In part, this book starts a journey of thinking differently about IPC and offers both stimulation and some innovative solutions going forward.

Leadership, culture, marketing, matters of justice, neuroscience and patient and family perspectives are not traditionally the predominant themes that stand out in a book on IPC. Indeed the conventional focus of the specialty has been heavily weighted towards what can be considered technical, scientific matters – structural, organisational and policy-related aspects of healthcare-associated infection, grounded in microbiology. This book complements the science, it brings humanity to IPC, intended to make us think, pause for a second, step outside the technical and consider the social value of what we do every day. It is refreshing to see a shift in focus.

Therefore, while acknowledging that in order to provide the highest quality of prevention and care to patients it is important to base approaches and interventions in the hardest science available, in parallel we must continue to consider the holistic aspects of IPC, open our mind to new perspectives – challenge the status quo and increasingly give a stronger voice to those who receive healthcare, including those who suffer harm. This book is bold in attempting just that.

What I particularly like about this book is that it perfectly illustrates the diversity of IPC. A number of the authors have worked with me personally at the international level and are acknowledged experts in the field. Through this book, all of them bring experiences and reflections that could be described as a breath of fresh air. We hear from student nurses and lecturers, hospital managers and leaders, a paramedic, academics and patients and their families.

This book should be welcomed and applauded for trying to shake up our thinking and make us question how we think and what we normally do. I sincerely hope it inspires some of you to think differently and of course act differently in the quest to save people from the devastation of healthcare infection.

Professor Benedetta Allegranzi
Lead, Clean Care is Safer Care and Infection Control Programme
Service Delivery and Safety Department
World Health Organization
Geneva
July 2015

Foreword by Marilyn Cruickshank

Patients expect safe, high-quality healthcare and their expectations are generally fulfilled. However, far too many patients acquire an infection during their encounter with the health system.

Growing public awareness through the media and public reporting of infection rates have led to more urgent action on specific risks by policy makers seeking answers to previously rising infection rates. The growth of multi-resistant organisms within the health systems makes the need for action more urgent as the miracle of antibiotics as a panacea becomes less reliable. Resistance may occur within months of the release of a new antimicrobial, and resistance is outstripping drug discovery and the development of new antimicrobials. The world is now facing the very real possibility of a return to non-treatable infections, severe limitations on medical procedure and escalating healthcare costs. Complex medicine such as organ transplantation, neonatal survival, intensive care and complex surgery may no longer be viable rather than everyday occurrences should antimicrobial resistance gain a hold in our health systems.

There are many strategies available for health systems to reduce infections involving systematic, national responses to infection control, hand hygiene and antibiotic stewardship. Bringing together policy makers and clinicians has been found to contribute to successful outcomes in the implementation of change management programs in reducing infection.

Improvement in technology provides tools for those charged with preventing infections to look beyond some of the tried and true methods of infection prevention. Building design can enhance good practice by providing single rooms and bathrooms for hospitalised patients; minimising patient transfers especially in multi-patient wards can also have an impact on infection spread; sufficient nursing staff numbers can also contribute to infection prevention.

Leadership at all levels of the health system, from national to hospital and within the infection prevention team, must be one of the single most powerful mechanisms to achieving change within the healthcare system. The opening chapters of this publication provide the infection control practitioner with an insight into effecting change in their environment through good management practices and appreciating the value of true leadership qualities. Without effective management and leadership there can be no improvement.

Challenges to improvement are many, and not least is our inability to provide randomised controlled evidence for all our practice. Using a common sense approach which according to one of my close colleagues is not so common can also be fraught with difficulty.

The prevention and control of healthcare associated infections is an essential element of patient safety and is the responsibility of all who provide care for patients, not just the infection control team. Infections are no longer considered an acceptable complication but rather an adverse event. Although not all may be preventable, it is possible to significantly reduce the rates preventing pain and suffering in patients as well as freeing up valuable bed days and clinician time.

It is heartening and joyous to read through this publication, not focused on the technical aspects of infection prevention, but focused on other just as pertinent skills that will result in doing great work for patients.

Adj Professor Marilyn Cruickshank RN, PhD, FACN
Director, National Healthcare Associated Infection Program
Australian Commission on Safety and Quality in Health Care
Sydney, NSW
July 2015

Preface

The adoption of appropriate infection prevention and control practices remains a significant problem within not only medicine, health and social care but also within our wider society at a global level, despite there being a significant and growing evidence base indicating the impact of the right practices on patient outcomes. Yet, despite this, compliance with safe infection prevention and control policy, education and published information remains less than satisfactory and much to the potential detriment of ourselves, our colleagues and the general population. Further, much of the published literature, although acting as a consistent reminder to us all, in many ways simply regurgitates the same information on a consistent basis, which really does not serve to move things forward in a positive way.

With these points in mind, this book sets out to offer some new perceptions and different perspectives related to infection prevention and control that may not have previously been considered and, in some cases, may seem left of centre. This is a very deliberate attempt to challenge us all to consider the status quo and to stimulate fresh ideas about where the specialty goes next. In reading through each of the chapters you will see that they are very individualistic and offer some unique, challenging and in some cases moving perspectives with regard to how each of the chapter authors perceives infection prevention and control, and from backgrounds you might not necessarily expect.

Further, as you read through the various chapters you will see that not all are referenced or, for that matter, particularly academic in nature. With regard to this, we, the editors, felt that where perceptions and perspectives were concerned it is not always necessary to be overly academic, because, where some of the chapters are concerned, it has more to do with the humanity of what contributors have written. In reading through each of the chapters it is hoped that this book will provide you with the opportunity to reflect upon each contributor's perception and/or perspective, and we would ask that you will take each chapter on its own merits and allow the limits of your thinking to be challenged.

LEARNING OUTCOMES

In reading through the chapters of this book you will have the opportunity to:

- reflect upon a number of differing approaches to infection prevention and control
- consider what the future of the specialty might hold for specialists, educationalists, practitioners and the public
- reflect upon your own attitudes and beliefs in relation to infection prevention and control
- reflect on the potential to use skills developed in infection prevention and control within other areas of professional practice
- recognise the constant changes in healthcare delivery that require continuous ongoing development for not just infection prevention and control practitioners, but all those involved in the provision of healthcare, irrespective of their appointment or role.
- facilitate and empower yourself to challenge the status quo, push the limits of infection prevention and control thinking and to reflect upon conventional wisdom.

Paul Elliott, Julie Storr, Annette Jeanes
July 2015

NOTE FROM THE EDITORS

With regard to each of the chapters in this book, should you wish to offer comment on the content then it is requested that you contact the individual contributor(s) directly.

Further, within each of the chapters the contributors' thoughts are theirs and do not necessarily reflect those of the editors or other contributors.

About the editors

Paul Elliott commenced his initial nurse education in 1971 at Royal Air Force Hospital Ely. Following this, the first half of Paul's professional career was spent serving in the Royal Air Force, undertaking a variety of roles within acute, community settings, aeromedical evacuation and field deployments. Following retirement from the Royal Air Force in 1985, Paul spent a number of years within the National Health Service and in 1991 he moved into higher education, which is where his career has continued to develop. Paul's primary research interests centre on the psychological aspects of infection prevention and control, and he has a range of publications and conference papers within this area. With regard to his current appointment, Paul is a Senior Lecturer in Adult Nursing and Infection Control within the School of Nursing at Canterbury Christ Church University in Kent.

Julie Storr graduated as a nurse and health visitor from the University of Manchester in 1990. Julie worked as a clinical nurse before specialising in infection prevention and control at Scunthorpe and Goole Hospitals NHS Trust and then the Oxford Radcliffe Hospital NHS Trust. In 2002 she was invited to join the National Patient Safety Agency as Assistant Director of Infection Prevention and directed the award-winning clean**your**hands™ campaign. Based on this work, in 2005 she was asked to take a lead role with the World Health Organization (WHO) on its First Global Patient Safety Challenge, pilot testing the WHO Guidelines on Hand Hygiene in Health Care in South East Asia and Latin America. Since 2009 she has worked for WHO's African Partnerships for Patient Safety programme and more recently within its Service Delivery and Safety Team as part of the Ebola response and recovery effort in West Africa. Julie is a trained clinical hypnotherapist. She is on the steering group of the charity HIFA (Health Information for All) and is studying for a doctorate in public health (healthcare leadership and management) at Johns Hopkins Bloomberg School of Public Health, in Baltimore, Maryland. She is an external examiner at University College Cork. She sits on the editorial advisory board of the *Journal of Infection Prevention* and is currently a director of S3 Global.

Annette Jeanes is currently the Director of Infection Prevention and Control and Consultant Nurse Infection Control at University College London Hospitals. She has worked at several London hospitals in intensive care, infectious diseases, medicine and surgery. She has acted as an external advisor to a number of national groups and forums. Her current research focus is improving hand hygiene compliance monitoring and performance. Other areas of interest include infection control in sport, cleaning in healthcare, reducing infection in surgical wounds, and the value of motivation and leadership in healthcare.

List of contributors

Yogi Amin
BSc, MB, ChB, FRCA
Consultant in Neuro-Anaesthesia
and Neuro-Intensive Care, National
Hospital for Neurology and
Neurosurgery, University College
London Hospitals NHS Foundation
Trust
Honorary Senior Lecturer, The UCL
Institute of Neurology, University
College London

Taraneh Azizi
BSc (Hons), Operating Department
Practice, RODP (HCPC)
Student SIG Lead, Association for
Perioperative Practice
Royal United Hospitals Bath NHS Trust

Derek Butler
Chairman, MRSA Action UK
Professional Engineer Nuclear Industry
Engineer, Westinghouse Electric
Company

Nizam Damani
MBBS, MSc, PRCPath, FRCP1, CIC,
DipHIC
Associate Medical Director: Infection
Prevention and Control, Craigavon
Area Hospital, Northern Ireland

Tara Donnelly
Director – Quality, Efficiency and
Productivity Programme, University
College London Hospitals NHS
Foundation Trust

Harley Farmer
PhD, BVSc(Hons), BVBiol(Path),
MRCVS
Virologist and Chief Executive Officer,
NewGenn Limited

Dave Grewcock
Head of Education Research and
Development, University College
London Hospitals NHS Foundation
Trust

Aidan Halligan
MB, BCh, BAO, BA, MA, MD
Director of Education, University
College London Hospitals NHS
Foundation Trust
Chief of Safety, Brighton and Sussex
University Hospitals NHS Trust

Clare Hancock
MPharm, MRPS
Clinical Pharmacist, The Royal Surrey
County Hospital NHS Foundation
Trust

Graziella Kontkowski
Clostridium Difficile Support Group,
    London
info@cdiff-support.co.uk

Maryanne McGuckin
FSHEA
President, McGuckin Methods
    International (A Patient Safety
    Organization)
Lead author of Patient Empowerment
    section of WHO Guidelines on Hand
    Hygiene in Healthcare (2009) Patient
    Safety
Former faculty member, University of
    Pennsylvania

Sarah Pye
RGN, DN, BSc (Hons), MA,
    PGCLT(HE), MRCN
Senior Lecturer Practice Learning,
    School of Nursing, Canterbury Christ
    Church University, Kent

Debra Teasdale
MSc, PGCLT, BSc, RN
Dean of the Faculty of Health and
    Wellbeing, Canterbury Christ Church
    University, Kent

Paul Vigar
BSc (Hons), PGCLT (HE), MC Para,
    FHEA
Senior Lecturer, Paramedic Science,
    Canterbury Christ Church University,
    Kent
Paramedic Practitioner, South East Coast
    Ambulance Service NHS Foundation
    Trust

Acknowledgements

We would like to acknowledge and offer our thanks to:

- each of the contributors, for their chapters and for their understanding regarding the length of time it has taken to complete this book
- Katrina Hulme-Cross, Louise Crowe, Gillian Nineham and Jamie Etherington for their support and understanding with regard to the development of this book.

*For everyone, everywhere, who has been affected by
an infection that should never have happened*

PART I

Perspectives of infection prevention and control

CHAPTER 1

Motivation and leadership in infection prevention and control

....
Annette Jeanes

In infection prevention and control, practitioners are frequently expected to lead, initiate or facilitate improvements or changes. The motivation and leadership of people is often challenging, particularly when associated with improving practice. This is even more complicated when you need to influence managers and leaders. The purpose of this chapter is to explain some of the theories and concepts associated with motivation and leadership and to suggest how these may be used within this specialty.

THEORIES OF MOTIVATION

Kreitner[1] defined motivation as 'the psychological process that gives behaviour purpose and direction', while Bedeian[2] suggested it is 'the will to achieve'. In this chapter the term motivation is used to describe the force that makes individuals do what they do, or perhaps what makes some staff wash their hands while others do not!

In ancient history, workers, slaves and servants were simply expected to obey and do the work. Their motivation was based on a need to eat and survive. Motivation was therefore relatively simple. In the current day some managers still believe that it is simple and that they know what motivates their staff, but this is a complex and developing field. Motivational theories vary and there is little consensus.

One traditional view of motivation is that people require tight control in the workplace and respond to reward and punishment. This is often referred to as the 'carrot and stick' method of motivation. Reinforcement theory[3] is based on rewarding good behaviour and not rewarding behaviour that is not wanted. This method has frequently been used to train animals and has also been successful with humans; however, it is predictable and may in time dwindle in efficacy. It is the basis for awards- or prize-based systems and is used in performance management.

Frederick Winslow Taylor was an early pioneer in 'scientific management'; he believed people were motivated by pay and worked more efficiently if work was divided into a series of tasks.[4] Staff could be allocated a simple, specific task and be paid according to productivity. This approach was adopted widely in manufacturing industries – including Ford, where assembly lines led to greater efficiencies, although boredom with repetitive tasks caused job dissatisfaction.[5] In addition, although workers were paid more if they worked faster, this could lead to lay-offs, as fewer staff were required and there was a lack of overtime, which was a disincentive. This prompted conflict between managers and workers, and actions such as 'working to rule' developed in response.

Elton Mayo conducted what are now known as the 'Hawthorne studies'.[6] These studies demonstrated that employee behaviour is linked to attitudes and that rewards are not just monetary. It was concluded from this work that just being part of a study or being observed and monitored changed behaviour and could improve or change performance. The 'Hawthorne effect' is often used to explain the improvements in infection control performance noted while observation is taking place. A good example is the improvements identified in hand hygiene compliance while observational monitoring takes place.[7]

McGregor[8] believed that work was a natural requirement and that matching the developmental needs of individuals to organisational goals leads to optimal motivation and performance. In his 'x' and 'y' theory of management styles he argued that the 'x' type management style, which is autocratic and controlling, leads to poor results, while the 'y' type management style, which is participative, allows staff self-control and self-regulation, which in turn allows staff to develop and contribute more. Standardised and consistent infection control practice may be difficult to maintain and monitor in a self-regulated team if the team decides to do something different from everyone else; this may be challenging for infection control staff.

Herzberg[9] concluded that there are two elements to motivation. The first comprises 'hygiene' factors, which include environment, supervision, relationships with others and pay. These factors can demotivate if they are inadequate. The second element is related to job satisfaction and is termed 'motivational' factors – these include recognition and achievement. This has been compared to Maslow's hierarchy of needs theory,[10] which places the basic physiological needs of food and shelter at the base of the hierarchy, followed by safety, social, ego and self-actualisation at the top.

The 'motivational' factors can be misinterpreted as a rehash of the 'carrot and stick' approach but it is more complex, as individual motivation varies. If you need to ensure people do what you want, it is important to understand what motivates them to do a job and consistently do it well. Herzberg[9] argued that motivation accrued from monetary reward and was also associated with the recognition of value and achievement in the job. It can cause dissatisfaction if the pay is felt to be too little for the effort, but work has a purpose beyond earning money. Work can provide stimulation, responsibility, purpose and a structure to day-to-day life. It can provide a social network, and individuals become part of a group, which provides social and psychological support.

Vroom[11] suggested that individuals are motivated by outcomes. These were termed 'valence', 'expectancy' and 'instrumentality'; they drive effort, performance and reward, and they are shaped by individual beliefs and preferences. A healthcare worker could theoretically clean hands well and consistently because he or she believes it is an important part of infection prevention and that it contributes toward patient welfare (valence). The healthcare worker could put in extra time and effort because this would improve the standard of infection prevention achieved, which would be noted (expectancy) and which may lead to improved patient outcome and the associated kudos, recognition or promotion (instrumentality).

OTHER FACTORS THAT INFLUENCE MOTIVATION

Workplaces and work groups also have a role in motivation, as they provide a communication network and a cohesiveness that links the group. The core values are generally shared by peers and dissent is discouraged, as dissent undermines the dynamics of the group and the status quo. Peer pressure is an important motivating factor in changing behaviours and embedding changes. Generally, people respond to peer pressure and aim to be accepted by their peers. Groups may be unaware that they hold negative values and perceptions, and this may influence their ability to assimilate or evaluate change or initiatives objectively.[12] Alternatively, peer pressure can be a strong force in accepting changes or raising standards. There are many examples of peer pressure improving infection control compliance, including hand hygiene.[13]

Perceptions are also important and affect motivation, development and opportunities. The concept of the self-fulfilling prophesy or Pygmalion effect[14] is that if opportunities are given and people are treated appropriately, they have the potential to achieve a lot, but that subconscious cues and expectations influence the overall performance obtained. Therefore, an optimistic and positive approach to change in the right circumstances may have a positive motivational effect. There is also a danger that focusing energy on non-compliant, poorly performing staff may demotivate the compliant staff, who may feel overlooked in the presence of the prevalent negative expectation; this may be the case in many areas of infection control practice, including waste disposal, isolation practices, screening, sampling and cleaning.

Job satisfaction is an important indicator of how individuals feel about their job. If this can be improved it may lead to increased motivation and even productivity, although the correlation between job satisfaction and productivity is tenuous.[15] Job satisfaction may affect sickness and absence rates, contribute to staff turnover and affect behaviours of individuals within the organisation; however, it is affected by individual dispositions, characteristics and experiences.

To retain valued employees, some employers are now using approaches such as job sculpting.[16] This designs the job to meet the needs of the worker, using the principles of optimising production developed by Taylor.[4] Empowerment, autonomy, job enrichment, fulfilment and flexibility are all linked to increasing motivation. Developing and supporting an infection control link staff programme, for example, may lead to increased job satisfaction and motivation, as these staff are supported to develop a knowledge and skill set that may have a positive benefit.

Effective managers and leaders understand the value of motivation and use it judiciously. It is also important in infection prevention and control to understand the role of leadership and managers in change management.

LEADERSHIP AND MANAGEMENT

Leadership plays an important role in change management and service improvement. Leadership influences change and often manipulates and manages change.[17] There are many change management theories, but the classic original change model was developed by Lewin *et al.*[18] This three-stage model – unfreezing, changing and then refreezing– essentially prepared the worker for change (unfreeze), made the change (change) and then ensured the change became permanent (refreeze).

Another model commonly used is Kotter's[19] 8-step change model (*see* Figure 1.1), which begins with what has been described as a 'burning platform'. This sort of approach is used frequently in infection prevention and control strategies – for example, prevention of needlestick injuries, and reduction of the use of antibiotics.

The problem with models such as Kotter's is that they are leadership driven and can be coercive. This may affect job satisfaction and motivation, which may also lead to resistance to change. Consequently, the approach to leadership or style of leadership is an important factor in change management. It can be influenced by a number of factors, including experience, values, beliefs, preferences, ability, culture and norms, the environments and the situation.

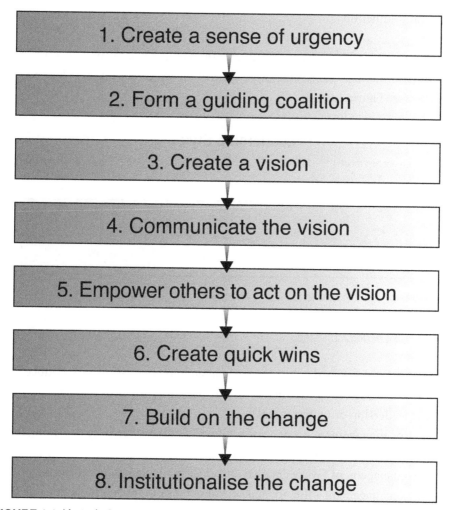

FIGURE 1.1 Kotter's 8-step change model[19]

LEADERSHIP STYLES

The classic leadership styles described by Lewin[18] are autocratic, democratic and laissez-faire or delegative. Each style has its own positive and negative aspects. There are also various types of leader:

● charismatic
● participative
● situational

- transactional
- transformational
- the quiet leader
- servant/authentic.

The style of leadership relates to the degree of managerial control. The less control the leader or manager exerts, the more control the worker or follower has, and the converse (*see* Figure 1.2).

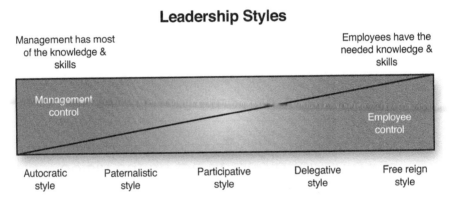

Leadership Styles

FIGURE 1.2 Leadership styles

A number of styles of leadership or management have been shown to produce poor outcomes, although they continue to occur:

- toxic leadership or management[20]
- post hoc management – a generally autocratic style, often only providing management after the event or in a crisis
- micromanagement – very detailed and close management and control
- seagull management – flies in, makes a lot of noise, craps on everything and then flies off again, leaving a big mess behind
- kipper management – a two-faced manager with different approaches for different situations
- the glory hog or user – takes the credit but does not do the work.

Many infection control practitioners will have encountered at least one of these examples.

The perpetuation of poor managers created by large organisations and by business schools has led to criticism. Sumantra Ghoshal stated: 'Asshole management is not inevitable.'[21] He observed:

It is interesting that a confluence of very diverse endeavours – that of economists to make the practice of management amoral, that of strategy and organisation theorists to make it scientific, and that of journalists and consultants to make it heroic – have collectively reinforced the rise of asshole management.[21]

Ghoshal argued that management should be a 'force for good' but that in the established and what he termed 'old style management' it was 'solutions first, people second', which led to an emphasis on the management of people to change.[21]

Axelrod[22] proposed that an alternative to leader-driven change is collaborative leadership. Key elements of collaborative leadership are engagement, relationships and democracy. It is based on the principles of honesty, transparency and trust.

The Enron and WorldCom scandals prompted a desire for leaders who could be trusted, and this led to the concept and publication of *Authentic Leadership* by Bill George.[23] The notion of 'authenticity' was already well established in counselling, psychotherapy and coaching. It is defined as being true to character, true to oneself; not living through a false image or false emotions that hide the real you, being genuine not a copy or clone.

Authentic leaders purport to know and live their values; they win people's trust by being who they are, not pretending to be someone else or living up to the expectations of others. Character development, inner leadership or self-mastery is crucial to becoming an authentic leader.

Elements of authentic leadership:

- being true to yourself in the way you work – no facade
- being motivated by a larger purpose (not by your ego)
- being prepared to make decisions that feel right and that fit your values – not decisions that are merely politically astute or designed to make you popular
- concentrating on achieving long-term sustainable results.[24]

Popular use of the term 'authentic leader' and modifications has blurred the definition, the main overlap being with 'servant leadership'.[25] The concept of 'a leader who serves' is well established, with one of the earliest references to servant leadership being Jesus Christ. Essentially, the concept is of a self-sacrificing leadership that prioritises the interests of the organisation and the well-being of workers.

There are number of problems with this type of leader in practice, such as 'How long will such a leader or hero last? How can you be sure that their motives and values are genuine? How do they accurately determine the best interests of organisation and workers? Isn't compromise a more sustainable solution?'

Organisational constraints and imperatives may not easily support authentic or servant leadership. Instead, the industrialisation of healthcare has promoted speed and efficiency, increasing standardisation of tasks and the use of technology. Control and consistency are important in this environment. It has been argued that this has led the rise of a managerial class that oversees a deskilled workforce in which division of labour is more common.[26] Examples in healthcare include nurses who have to be trained to give a flu vaccine because their jobs do not involve giving injections, staff who cannot use a manual blood pressure machine or thermometer, or staff who need a computer to calculate doses of drugs or provide a plan of care.

MANAGEMENT VERSUS LEADERSHIP

Kotter[27] argued that the function of management is homeostasis and to keep the system functioning constantly. Part of this process is control, and another part is having a target or objective. Management systems are often designed to consistently deliver a target, to monitor the system and act when the target is at risk; an example is the monitoring and managing of budgets and finances.

The control and planning required by managers may be problematic in infection control, as new microorganisms and outbreaks of infections are often unpredictable and infections prevented are not noticed. In addition, the work required by infection control staff is dependent on those who deliver the care or service. To deliver improvements in practice, management and control of behaviours is usually essential at the point of delivery, but the managerial pressure to perform or meet targets is often focused on the infection control practitioners.

Managers may offer rewards for improved performance but require control and constancy. Kotter argues that leadership is different, as it uses motivational or inspirational processes to energise by 'satisfying basic human needs: achievement, belonging, recognition, self-esteem, a sense of control over one's life, and living up to one's ideals'.[27] He also argues that motivating people for a short time is easy, particularly in a crisis, but that motivating them long term takes planning and commitment.

Leadership and management are linked but they are not the same thing. Bennis[28] composed a list of the differences:
- The manager administers; the leader innovates.
- The manager is a copy; the leader is an original.
- The manager maintains; the leader develops.
- The manager focuses on systems and structure; the leader focuses on people.

- The manager relies on control; the leader inspires trust.
- The manager has a short-range view; the leader has a long-range perspective.
- The manager asks how and when; the leader asks what and why.
- The manager has his or her eye always on the bottom line; the leader's eye is on the horizon.
- The manager imitates; the leader originates.
- The manager accepts the status quo; the leader challenges it.
- The manager is the classic good soldier; the leader is his or her own person.
- The manager does things right; the leader does the right thing.

Although twenty-first-century healthcare has its emphasis on efficiency, healthcare workers are not just part of a machine. The value of people is frequently associated with the knowledge and experience they bring to the job. To get the best from people they need to be nurtured.

Peter Drucker[29] wrote of the rise of the knowledge worker and how the requirement was now less to manage people. 'The task is to lead people. And the goal is to make productive the specific strengths and knowledge of every individual.'[30] One of the ways this has been done is by empowerment.

EMPOWERMENT

Empowered staff are able to make decisions, are given responsibility and can decide how to undertake the work they do. This increases motivation, engagement and job satisfaction. The quality of the service delivered may improve, as the staff are more likely to accept ownership and responsibility for outcomes.

This does not occur in a vacuum and requires an organisational culture, leadership and management support system to facilitate and support empowered workers. To succeed it also requires a skilled and knowledgeable workforce with a clear understanding of the organisation's objectives and values.

In some organisations this has been taken further, with self-managed teams shown to be more effective than traditionally managed teams.[31] These teams make decisions and adopt approaches that fit their circumstances and which work.

Unfortunately, in the current era of bundles of evidence-based practice and numerous imposed guidelines, it has become increasingly unlikely that infection control practitioners will be encouraged to take approaches that are not in line with standard practice. The imposition of innovations and interventions that have been found useful in other organisations and situation is likely to continue, even though they may not work elsewhere.

However, there are opportunities to adapt rather than blindly adopt imposed initiatives. Empowering staff to make local adaptations and variations is likely to be more effective than imposing and dictating. The role of infection prevention and control practitioners is to ensure the staff have the education training and support to make the adaptations with confidence and to allow them to own the initiative and, it is to be hoped, the associated kudos.

CONCLUSION

This chapter has provided some explanation and detail of the theories and issues of motivation and leadership. Understanding motivation is important in effectively leading and managing or working with leaders and managers. It can improve the effectiveness of infection prevention and control practitioners and the sustainability of initiatives.

It is essential that you communicate effectively, simply and clearly. What is your goal? What is the plan? Who do you need to influence? This may mean that you have to adapt your style and methods according to the audience, situation or opportunity. It is also important to ensure that you adapt your approach based on your experience and by listening or learning from others.

Teamwork, encouraging others and empowering others are also crucial factors. Infection prevention and control is largely about getting others to do things the right way. This relies on them being motivated and engaged to do it consistently while you are not there. This may be hard to achieve, as what motivates and engages staff may vary from one organisation, team or individual to another.

Finally, integrity, reliability, stability, honesty and humility as a leader, manager, team member or individual are important. Courage is crucial, as the potential difficulties encountered in this specialty cannot be understated. In particular when you have to speak out in identifying poor practice or care, communicate with difficult managers or admit to an error. The way you behave and respond affects those you interact with, and subsequently the safety and satisfaction of patients.

REFERENCES
1. Kreitner R. *Management.* 6th ed. Boston, MA: Houghton Mifflin; 1995.
2. Bedeian AG. *Management.* 3rd ed. New York, NY: Dryden Press; 1993.
3. Skinner BF. *Science and Human Behavior.* New York, NY: The Free Press; 1953.
4. Taylor FW. *Principles of Scientific Management.* New York, NY: Harper & Brothers; 1911.
5. Batchelor R. *Henry Ford, Mass Production, Modernism and Design.* Trowbridge: Redwood Books; 1994.

6. Mayo GE. *The Human Problems of an Industrial Civilization*. Reprint ed. London: Routledge; 2003.
7. Eckmanns T, Bessert J, Behnke M, *et al.* Compliance with antiseptic hand rub use in intensive care units: the Hawthorne effect. *Infect Control Hosp Epidemiol.* 2006; **27**(9): 931–4.
8. McGregor D. *The Human Side of Enterprise*. New York, NY: McGraw-Hill; 1960.
9. Herzberg FI. One more time: how do you motivate employees? *Harv Bus Rev.* 1987; **65**(5): 109–20.
10. Maslow AH. A theory of human motivation. *Psychol Rev.* 1943; **50**(4): 370–96.
11. Vroom VH. *Work and Motivation*. New York, NY: John Wiley & Sons; 1964.
12. Estlund C. *Working Together: how workplace bonds strengthen a diverse democracy*. New York, NY: Oxford University Press; 2003.
13. Haessler S, Bhagavan A, Kleppel R, *et al.* Getting doctors to clean their hands: lead the followers. *BMJ Qual Saf.* 2012; **21**(6): 499–502.
14. Rosenthal R, Jacobson L. *Pygmalion in the Classroom: teacher expectation and pupils' intellectual development*. New York, NY: Rinehart & Winston; 1968.
15. Judge TA, Thoresen CJ, Bono JE, *et al.* The job satisfaction-job performance relationship: a qualitative and quantitative review. *Psychol Bull.* 2001; **127**(3): 376–407.
16. Butler T, Waldroop J. Job sculpting: the art of retaining your best people. *Harv Bus Rev.* 1999; **77**(5): 144–52.
17. Ovretveit J. Improvement leaders: what do they and should they do? A summary of a review of research. *Qual Saf Health Care.* 2010; **19**(6): 490–2.
18. Lewin K, Lippitt R, White RK. Patterns of aggressive behavior in experimentally created social climates. *J Soc Psychol.* 1939; **10**: 271–301.
19. Kotter JP. *Leading Change*. Boston, MA: Harvard Business School Press; 1996.
20. Kets de Vries MF. Coaching the toxic leader. *Harv Bus Rev.* 2014; **92**(4): 100–9.
21. Birkinshaw J, Piramal G. *Sumantra Ghoshal on Management: a force for good*. King's Lynn, UK: Prentice Hall; 2005.
22. Axelrod R. *The Evolution of Cooperation*. Revised ed. New York, NY: Perseus Books; 2006.
23. George W. *Authentic Leadership: rediscovering the secrets to creating lasting value*. San Francisco, CA: Jossey-Bass; 2003.
24. George W, McLean A, Craig N. *Finding Your True North: a personal guide*. Chichester: Jossey-Bass; 2008.
25. Greenleaf RK. *Servant Leadership*. New York, NY: Paulist Press; 1977.
26. Rastegar DA. Health care becomes an industry. *Ann Fam Med.* 2004; **2**(1): 79–83.
27. Kotter JP. *A Force for Change: how leadership differs from management*. New York, NY: The Free Press; 1990.
28. Bennis W. *On Becoming a Leader*. Cambridge, MA: Perseus Books; 1989.
29. Drucker PF. *The Landmarks of Tomorrow*. New York, NY: Harper & Brothers; 1959.
30. Drucker PF. *Management Challenges for the 21st Century*. New York, NY: HarperCollins; 2001.
31. Cohen SG, Ledford GE Jr. The effectiveness of self-managing teams: a quasi-experiment. *Hum Relat.* 1994; **47**(1): 13–43.

CHAPTER 2

Just infection prevention and control

....

Julie Storr

Information giving and anxiety reduction should be fundamental parts of nursing.[1]

INTRODUCTION

Over 20 years ago, a conversation was stimulated on the challenges of moving away from outdated nursing procedures that are based on myths and consist of ritualistic behaviour and which are carried out by healthcare practitioners (nurses) without thinking and insight.[1] This chapter resumes the conversation in the present day, through an infection prevention and control lens. It explores what, if any, are the present-day myths and rituals in modern healthcare that are carried out in the name of infection prevention and control, alongside practices that have become accepted as the norm. Most important, it considers the unintended consequences that such myths and misconceptions can have, particularly in terms of injustice, inequity, ethics and psychological harm. It calls for action now where warranted to stop injustice, to refocus on activities that are safe, evidence informed, patient focused and, ultimately, sensible. It subsequently highlights the need to build capacity and capability across healthcare such that insight into the consequences of what is carried out in the name of infection control is readdressed, posing the question: 'What can we do better to ensure justice for infection prevention in the name of patient safety?' This chapter culminates in a number of proposed actions, including a healthcare worker training revolution, research on the impact of redundant or unnecessary practices on the psychological health of patients, a 'consumer or future patient' awareness-raising campaign – driven by policy and supported by informed media – and infection prevention and control strategies that are focused on halting microbial transmission and subsequent harm from a holistic, rights-based perspective that takes account of dignity, ethics, humanity and justice.

Hospital workers exercise care through a network of practices and fundamental beliefs that are largely taken for granted. This author emphasises the 'embodied know-how that goes into a surgeon's operations, or into the touch of the doctor or nurse when examining a patient' – care described as grounded in skilful micropractices that healthcare workers have absorbed and carry out without freshly thinking them through on each occasion. It is only when aspects of practice become problematic that they are raised for debate and can be changed.[2]

For a long time infection prevention and control has been focused on the impact of microbes on the health and well-being of patients, and on how practices control the spread of these microbes. Is it now perhaps the moment to consider the patient-related impact of some of the micro- and macro-practices that are in place in the name of halting transmission; some of the 'problems' associated with these; and to call time on those that at least might be unnecessary and at worst might actually be harmful.

BOX 2.1 A personal reflection

My first recollection of infection control, as it was then described, was during the last century – the 1980s to be precise, and my first ward placement as a student nurse. I recall being told in no uncertain terms and most seriously by a healthcare assistant that on no account must I use talcum powder when assisting a patient with activities of daily living, because of the infection hazard it presented. Whether this was rooted in scientific evidence I never got to know, because I accepted it on its face value as a fact.

The account described in Box 2.1 is reflective of a pattern that has permeated the rest of my career, initially in nursing and more recently healthcare.

Similar 'advice' continues to be heard to this day, ranging from a dentist who explained that the regulators instructed him to take a poster off the ceiling (it was intended to be a distraction to the anxious dental patient) because it presented an infection risk, to a nurse who explained medicine carts were no longer used for the same reason. Ties, watches, sleeves, flowers, Christmas decorations, bed-sitters – all frowned on in the name of infection prevention. Some of the frowning might well be justifiable, and while talcum powder and Christmas decorations might not have a significant effect on recovery or the psychological status of a patient, some of the practices we do (some for no sound reason) in the name of infection prevention and control can and do have consequences, which range from low-level annoyance through to heightened anxiety levels of patients and their families. The negative consequences, not of microbes but of the prevention and control mechanisms we employ, have surprisingly generated little debate in the academic literature. This chapter is intended to stimulate a new debate.

While much of infection prevention is evidence informed (or is increasingly so), this chapter is predicated on the acceptance that some of the things we do under the guise of preventing infection are based in mythology, some ritualistic and some plain nonsense. Everything addressed in the next few pages can be challenged, disputed and argued against, and, as a progressive infection preventionist, I welcome such discourse. This chapter is intended to push the healthcare community to revisit what we do in the name of stopping infection from occurring and/or spreading. Exploring the extent of this problem, if it exists, and its impact on patients will form an important contribution to a patient-focused approach to infection prevention and the pursuit of care and treatment that is patient-centred as well as concerned with the important matter of risk reduction. Healthcare teams that interact with patients 24 hours a day must be empowered to critique, understand and apply good science as well as to know when to consign myths and injustices to Room 101.

This chapter will explore:

- unintended consequences of (unnecessary) patient isolation – actions that ignore cognitive well-being and contribute to both under- and over-compliance of necessary infection control practices such as the right times for hand hygiene
- implementation of policies and practices that have no grounding in infection prevention evidence or logic (i.e. related to uniforms, buckles, beds, ties, patient chairs, toys, visitors, and so on)
- the impact of misunderstanding the dynamics of microbial spread at the patient bedside and therefore foregoing some important patient interactions, such as a comforting touch
- losing sight of the human being, the person beneath the patient, including risk communication and its impact on anxiety levels.

Martin Luther King Jr has been credited with the statement: 'Of all the forms of inequality, injustice in health care is the most shocking and inhumane'.[3,4]* A number of infection prevention and control practices grounded in myth have the potential to result in and perpetuate injustice in modern healthcare, an issue that must be addressed for patient well-being. Examples are not too hard to find. In the English National Health Service at the time of writing there continue to exist hospitals that ban visitors during outbreaks of norovirus, using the infection prevention and control argument in its defence; this is, in fact, counter to national guidance that, while discouraging social visitors, cites 'operational expedience' rather than infection control as its rationale. Yet other National Health Service organisations are considering the use of Skype and FaceTime as a means of communication between patients and visitors when visiting is restricted because of infection risks.

BOX 2.2 Some questions

Before reading further, consider the following: How much investment, time and lobbying has gone into strengthening surveillance – really high-quality surveillance that has been proven to contribute to reduction in healthcare-associated infection? How much investment is put into building high-quality, competent practitioners who are skilled in epidemiology? How much pressure is there for hospitals to undertake surveillance across the range of common healthcare-associated infections? How much surveillance is mandatory? Contrast this with the amount of effort and zeal that many in healthcare, including at the policy level, put into 'bare below the elbows', auditing of commodes, and deep cleaning? What drove the latter focus on politically motivated edicts and what prevents the former investment on interventions that are evidence-informed? Is this, in the end, an injustice?

SETTING THE SCENE

There seems to be something very strange going on. Is it all in the interests of being seen to be doing something very noticeable about the worrying levels of hospital based infections, however ineffective and otherwise disruptive.[5]

---

* The Washington State Commission on African American Affairs reports that Martin Luther King Jr made this statement on 25 March 1966, at the Second National Convention of the Medical Committee for Human Rights.

You don't have to look too hard in the published and grey literature to find a plethora of examples of the zealous application of practices in the name of infection prevention and control. What emerges from many of these examples is a trade-off between the need to prevent harm (usually, but not always, to patients or other patients in the vicinity) and the need to maximise the health and well-being of individual patients, including physical and psychosocial well-being.

A number of these issues are described perfectly in a blog post exploring whether well-minded infection control procedures are in fact subverted.[6] Within the blog it is suggested that many infection control procedures, with their origins in the maintenance of patient safety, have become routinised into our mindset and detached from their original purpose. The banning of flowers, which thankfully no longer seems all-pervasive from an infection control perspective, is used to illustrate the point. There is no evidence that flowers pose a risk of infection; however, as the author states, the maintenance, arrangement and emptying of vases may be seen as a burden to already busy staff, and the risk of spillage of water an unwanted side issue. Rather than using these justifications, the infection control agenda added a sense of legitimacy and a kickback to justify the exclusion of flowers from general wards. Similar illustrations are used that include toys and magazines in communal areas and restrictions on the number of visitors. In some instances infection control has taken on a social role and become a means of control, or even a pointless exercise, rather than an evidence-based practice.

Iona Heath,[5] quoted at the start of this section, summarised some of the issues in an article. She described the prohibition in modern healthcare of sitting on a patient's bed, in the name of infection control. The article presents a compelling account of the benefits, as she perceives it, to patients when doctors are permitted to sit on a bed during an encounter. Heath[5] describes such interactions as precious and, alarmingly, suggests that this ban on bed-sitters seems to be imposed even when patients are dying. She suggests that infection control specialists enforcing such approaches lack humanity and common sense, and she cites the national evidence-based guidelines on infection prevention and control as being devoid of any mention of bed-sitting (or flowers – an issue previously addressed by Heath[5] in the *BMJ*). Her default assumption is that there is no evidence for such a rule. Heath[5] concludes by returning us to the issue of humanity and calls for bed-sitting (and flowers) to be freely permitted unless there is robust evidence to deter these 'elements of home' from penetrating hospitals and improving patient well-being.

> Patients consistently estimate that they have been given more time when the doctor sits down rather than stands.[5]

It seems that considering infection through the narrow chink of a microscope lens could contribute to some of the challenges described here. These brief examples suggest a problem illustrative of misguided thinking on what's right and wrong, influenced by a lack of insight, misapplication of knowledge or, indeed, absence of sound knowledge, and a silent infection prevention and control community that needs to shout much louder if it is to be part of the solution and not a contributor to the problem. The media undoubtedly play a role, as evidenced in a review of the drivers and influencers of the media coverage of meticillin-resistant *Staphylococcus aureus* (MRSA) in the early to mid 2000s.[7] The authors concluded that the media played a powerful role in driving policy away from scientific evidence and toward popular, 'common-sense' solutions, and in addition the authors touched on the weaknesses in the scientific community, including professional bodies, in their inability to penetrate the media machine with counterarguments.

So far, this chapter has provided two anecdotal examples to illustrate that there may be a problem. Does the scientific literature shed any more light on the subject?

HUMANITY, ETHICS, RIGHTS AND CONSEQUENCES

This section focuses on a snapshot of the literature that highlights the potential injustices; it does not aim to present a full literature review balancing these points with the benefits of infection prevention and control measures, as these are freely available in many other documents. The key point being posed is that these measures are being applied separately from other patient care needs.

Considering justice in infection control from an ethical standpoint draws out the important point that most infection prevention professionals enter the specialty from a clinical medicine background – one where the welfare of individual patients trumps broader social concerns – and this can result in infection control measures infringing on individual rights and liberties.[8] Examples cited include surveillance, isolation precautions and antimicrobial prudence. In terms of the impact of infection prevention practices, patient isolation has received the greatest attention. Isolation undoubtedly serves a purpose in helping to control the spread of some microorganisms. However, there is some documented work that reports the isolation of patients and subsequent 'barrier' precautions can lead to fewer bedside visits by doctors and nurses and thereby resultant negative psychological impact on the patient, as well as poorer perceived satisfaction with treatment.[9]

A recent systematic review aimed to determine whether contact isolation leads to psychological or physical problems for patients.[10] The authors looked at 16 studies on the impact of isolation on the mental well-being of patients, patient satisfaction, patient safety or time spent by healthcare workers in direct patient care using validated tools scoring for levels of anxiety and depression. Their findings conclude that isolation has a negative impact on the mental well-being and behaviour of patients, including higher scores for depression, anxiety and anger among isolated patients. The literature revealed that healthcare workers spent less time with patients in isolation and that patient satisfaction was adversely affected, particularly influenced by the extent to which patients were kept informed of their healthcare. Patient safety was also negatively affected, although this has been contended in other studies, and the review found an eightfold increase in adverse events. The authors suggest that patient education may be an important step to mitigate the adverse psychological effects of isolation. However, the review did not consider patient information within the context of an empowered, well-educated and well-informed health workforce.

More recently, as part of a doctoral thesis, Parker[11] synthesised eight qualitative research studies focused on patients' experiences of healthcare-associated infections. The findings follow a similar pattern to that already outlined – experience was largely negative, psychological needs were often overlooked and fear, worry, stress and guilt were common features of the patient's experience. The patient experience was exacerbated by poor information-giving by staff, based on preconceptions and assumptions. Parker[11] describes the negative experience as resulting in a 'double iatrogenic effect' on the patient. The issue of poor information-giving predicated on limitations in staff knowledge and competence in the field is not explored in any detail.

It seems logical from this brief review of the literature that isolation is applied only when absolutely necessary for patient safety and that healthcare workers are aware of its potentially negative side effects.

What emerges from much of the literature is the need for a philosophical and ethical debate focused on the complexity that is infection prevention and control, and its practices that are ubiquitous and often never challenged. Many of the academic papers cited here focus on issues of justice, individual human rights, freedom of movement, the greater good of society and citizenship. Bryan and colleagues,[8] in particular, suggest that national guidelines and regulations sometimes fail to offer tidy solutions to infection prevention and control problems. Therefore, what is needed is a decision-making process that includes a careful review of the facts, values and external factors (such as guidelines) and an awareness of relevant ethical frameworks.

Healthcare-associated infection has also been considered from a patient rights perspective, addressing respect for human dignity, and this adds an interesting dimension to the debate.[12] Millar[12] describes the universality of human rights, particularly for citizens unable to advocate for themselves, and considers the isolation of patients as a potential breach of the right to dignity and respect. Millar[12] further discusses control strategies for MRSA and suggests that such measures operate at the interface between public health and the promotion of public good, and the care of individual patients – something that creates a tension within healthcare. Millar[12] proposes that historically there has been an acceptance by patients of the many actions that are taken to prevent and control healthcare-associated infection; however, by considering issues of patient rights, it becomes a matter of importance to be able to justify the measures taken.

> If patient rights are to be over-ridden, patients and the public might reasonably expect there to be transparent and explicit reasons, preferably supported not only by professional and expert opinion of the evidence but also consensus agreement with patients and the public.[12]

More recently, a World Health Organization Europe document[13] considered the important aspect of patient rights in relation to patient safety. Its chief focus is on the right to safe healthcare and it explores patient empowerment as one component of this, in relation to a number of safety-related areas including hand hygiene improvement. It does not concern itself with rights in relation to the unintended consequences of patient safety interventions.

In terms of a possible resolution of the conflicts identified in this chapter, Stelfox and colleagues[9] call for multicomponent interventions that are implemented in the name of patient safety, and this applies to many of the infection prevention practices described so far – particularly isolation – to have their individual parts examined to determine whether all elements are essential. They suggest that it might be possible to 'disentangle' which isolation policy components are most important for infection control and which may be most harmful to the isolated patient. They further call for individualisation, citing that patients who experience the most negative effects of isolation may not be those who present the greatest risk of microbial transmission. These authors discuss the interdependence of individual patient characteristics, clinician factors, environmental constraints and organisational culture as key influencers of patient safety.

MRSA was described in a recent paper as 'the infectious stigma of our time',[14] the paper challenging the reader to consider some of the things undertaken in the name of infection prevention guidelines. Here are some examples of practices uncovered during a reflective analysis of MRSA guideline application in Norway:

- older patients with dementia isolated for long periods

- patients denied access to a GP practice and had their consultation in a car park
- new employees made to stand naked and be examined for skin lesions.

The authors understandably ask the question, 'Oh God, what are we doing?' They consider the dichotomy of guideline implementation and an appreciation of the ethical dilemmas this can raise.

> We isolate people as if they have highly contagious TB [tuberculosis], but they may be as 'healthy' as persons with HIV [human immunodeficiency virus].[14]

These authors go on to suggest that MRSA, in particular, is unique in that it can result in the isolation of carriers who do not have clinical disease. This isolation can result in feelings of anxiety and powerlessness, and this is further compounded because often the time period for isolation is not well defined. The use of personal protective equipment, in some instances, by visitors can result in fewer visits by loved ones and in social deprivation. The authors conclude by calling for more emphasis on ethics within guidelines such as those designed to limit transmission of MRSA; at the very least they should contain an explicit ethical argument. The authors further suggest that we have failed to learn the lessons from the era of HIV, when in an attempt to prevent stigmatisation, universal precautions were introduced. The authors call for healthcare workers not to rely on passive conveyance of the measures suggested in guidelines, but rather to reflect on possible actions, particularly the ethical considerations and implications of the guidelines on patients and relatives.[14]

It seems that, increasingly, the research community is beginning to challenge some of the historic approaches to infection prevention and control. Spence and colleagues[15] describe how they have ceased to apply contact precautions within their 285-bed hospital in the United States for patients asymptomatically colonised with MRSA, with no noticeable impact on transmission. However, as with many hospitals in the United States, all patients in this 285-bed hospital have their own room; this is not the case at present in the United Kingdom.

Recently, there have also been some fresh voices and opinions heard on this topic, highlighted through the power that is social media, with eminent infectious disease physicians and epidemiologists in the United States using their blog post* to share thoughts on topics such as 'Why I Hate Contact Precautions' and 'Let Me

---

* haicontroversies.blogspot.com

BOX 2.3 Reflective exercise – the case for or against

Consider the following scenarios.

- Visitors of a patient isolated because of a resistant organism are instructed to wear gloves and a plastic apron on entry to the room and for the duration of their visit
- A postpartum woman being treated for a breast abscess due to MRSA is told she is not allowed to visit her infant in the busy neonatal intensive care unit in which MRSA has not yet emerged as a significant problem (adapted from Bryan et al.[8])
- A sign outside the entrance to a ward instructing visitors not to take flowers onto the ward
- A recommendation is made in a report of 'failing hospitals' for the health service to consider introducing Skype and FaceTime for patients in isolation, to minimise visitors
- A nurse in a nursing uniform, with a coat, the uniform looks clean and smart, enters a supermarket; the manager of the shop emails the manager of the local hospital to complain, citing risk of infection as a concern
- A report from a regulatory body that has undertaken a review of what are considered 'failing hospitals' criticises the infection prevention and control team because of a number of noticeable breaches of best practice, including one example of nurses wearing buckles
- An elevator in a large teaching hospital instructs all visitors to clean their hands as they enter a ward

For each scenario, try to answer the following three questions:

1. What is the key risk and who is it a risk to?
2. How strong, if at all, do you think the evidence behind the infection prevention and control measures is?
3. What might be the unintended consequences of the measures, and to whom?

If the measures are justified, in your opinion, how might the unintended consequences be lessened?

Hate on Contact Precautions Some More'. These challenging discussions must be welcomed and the role of social media explored further as a catalyst for change. The reflective exercises in Box 2.3 invite the reader to consider his or her own controversies and present a number of probing questions.

WHAT WE CAN DO MOVING FORWARD

This chapter has focused on aspects of infection prevention and control that may have unintended consequences and which could be described as perpetuating injustice for patients. A key focus has been on the impact of isolation on a patient's cognitive well-being, but there are other examples of practices implemented in the name of infection prevention, practices where the consequences have so far evaded academic scrutiny and have largely bypassed any sort of challenge or healthy debate. These are summarised in the following list – this list is certainly not exhaustive, but it aims to prompt action now where warranted to help stop injustice, and to refocus on activities that are safe, evidence informed, patient focused and, ultimately, sensible.

- Patient isolation only when absolutely necessary for patient safety, taking heed of the existing research (i.e. what we already know) about the psychological impact of isolation and contact precautions
- Compassion-informed risk communication when addressing infection/colonisation in patients, making the best use of all available skills and resources
- The development of a competent infection prevention-informed workforce and a gigantic leap forward in capacity building at the undergraduate and postgraduate level, driven by competent specialist practitioners
- Informed leadership, policymakers and regulators across every level of healthcare who promote the right culture for infection prevention
- An informed media ready to listen to a strong, credible and convincing scientific community
- The use of digital social media to promote the right messages
- Revisiting of the learning from HIV and universal precautions and consideration of the ethical argument for all infection prevention interventions
- Refocusing on evidence base and surveillance, and the impact of recommendations and data on behaviour
- Empowering patients and consumers – patient education and information on the rationale for everything undertaken in the name of infection prevention and control

And there are other aspects that should at least be considered now:
- research that looks beyond the impact of the germs, exploring the impact of redundant or unnecessary practices on the psychological health of patients
- a revolution in healthcare worker training, and bold moves to change how we approach this, with the goal of true capacity building and true behaviour change
- revised infection prevention and control strategies that are focused on halting microbial transmission and subsequent harm from a holistic, rights-based perspective that takes account of dignity, ethics, humanity and justice.

CONCLUSION

The topics that have been touched on in this chapter show that a number of practices appear to have lost sight of the person beneath the patient, and some of them have undoubtedly lost sight of the dynamics of spread of microbes at the bedside that can lead to patient harm. Based on what we now know in the twenty-first century, this chapter calls for all those working in healthcare to refocus on what infection prevention and control stands for, perhaps to redefine the specialty, and certainly to ensure that the practices carried out in its name never lose sight of the patient and his or her family. This requires strong, informed leadership to generate the right cultural milieu and a cadre of bold, progressive and pragmatic healthcare personnel to drive a new agenda.

Bryan and colleagues[8] introduce the notion of practical wisdom and love as key virtues for competence and caring, and that all healthcare workers, including infection preventionists and hospital epidemiologists, need *practical wisdom* to guide them in decision making in the face of uncertainty, to seek a balance between individual rights and the common good; *temperance* to seek restraint in the use of healthcare resources; and *courage* to engage busy and politically powerful physicians and administrators in dialogue. In conclusion, this chapter calls for an immediate cessation of the perpetuation of any injustice that is introduced or promoted in the name of infection prevention and control.

Additionally, infection prevention practitioners need to lead by standing up and denouncing anything that contributes minimally to patient safety and emerge as the credible, respected champions of logic, patient-centred care and safety. In the achievement of an exemplar culture of infection prevention and control, there is a need to win the hearts and minds of clinicians and managers. Much progress has been made but the need remains to strive for the right balance between risk, human rights and human wrongs. This is a challenge to all involved in healthcare and will involve a multifaceted approach. Infection preventionists should be blazing the trail, but it is the doctor, the nurse, the student, the porter, the domestic assistant and all those who exercise care through what Farrands[2] described as the network of practices and fundamental beliefs that are largely taken for granted. These are the workers who touch the lives of patients every day. Each interaction should be safe and sound, just and sensible, and not influenced in any way by myths and rituals that have the potential to cause harm.

REFERENCES

1. Walsh M, Ford P. *Nursing Rituals, Research and Rational Actions*. Oxford: Heinemann; 1989.
2. Farrands R. Hospitals: human bodies? *RSA Journal*. Summer 2013; **159**(5554): 22–3.
3. Moore A. *Tracking Down Martin Luther King, Jr.'s Words on Health Care*. HuffingtonPost. com; 2013 Jan 18, updated 2013 Mar 20. Available at: www.huffingtonpost.com/amanda-moore/martin-luther-king-health-care_b_2506393.html (accessed 15 December 2014).
4. Washington State Commission on African American Affairs. *Health Disparities: health gap reflects history of racism and mistrust*. Olympia, WA: Washington State Commission on African American Affairs; n.d. Available at: www.caa.wa.gov/priorities/health/HealthDisparities.shtml (accessed 15 December 2014).
5. Heath I. Do not sit on the bed. *BMJ*. 2010; **340**: c1478.
6. Lilford R. *Richard Lilford's Friday Blog: can well-minded infection control procedures be subverted?* 2012 Dec 7. Available at: richardlilfordsfridayblog.wordpress.com/2012/12/07/can-well-minded-infection-control-procedures-be-subverted/ (accessed 9 March 2013).
7. Boyce T, Murray E, Holmes A. What are the drivers of the UK media coverage of meticillin-resistant *Staphylococcus aureus*, the inter-relationships and relative influences? *J Hosp Infect*. 2009; **73**(4): 400–7.
8. Bryan CS, Call TJ, Elliott KC. The ethics of infection control: philosophical frameworks. *Infect Control Hosp Epidemiol*. 2007; **28**(9): 1077–84.
9. Stelfox HT, Bates DW, Redelmeier DA. Safety of patients isolated for infection control. *JAMA*. 2003; **290**(14): 1899–905.
10. Abad C, Fearday A, Safdar N. Adverse effects of isolation in hospitalised patients: a systematic review. *J Hosp Infect*. 2010; **76**(2): 97–102.
11. Parker N. *The Psychological Impact of Nosocomial Infection: a phenomenological investigation of patients' experiences of* Clostridium difficile [dissertation]. Leicester: University of Leicester; 2011.
12. Millar M. Patient rights and healthcare-associated infection. *J Hosp Infect*. 2011; **79**(2): 99–102.
13. World Health Organization (WHO). *Exploring Patient Participation in Reducing Health-Care-Related Safety Risks*. Copenhagen: WHO Regional Office for Europe; 2013.
14. Braut GS, Holt J. Meticillin-resistant *Staphylococcus aureus* infection – the infectious stigma of our time? *J Hosp Infect*. 2011; **77**(2): 148–52.
15. Spence MR, Dammel T, Courser S. Contact precautions for methicillin-resistant *Staphylococcus aureus* colonization: costly and unnecessary. *Am J Infect Control*. 2012; **40**(6): 535–8.

CHAPTER 3

Leadership, quality, efficiency and productivity in infection control

. . . .

Tara Donnelly

STONE SOUP

There is a tale told in many traditions of a wandering peasant woman who arrives in a village to find a community struck by deep poverty and famine. She arrives in the village square, takes a smooth stone from her apron pocket and claims it has magical properties such that she is able to make delicious soup from it. A crowd develops and the villagers look on with scepticism, as she asks for the largest cauldron they have to be filled with water and placed on a fire. Nonetheless, they bring it to her. She drops in the stone and then tastes the soup, declaring it good, but that it would taste even better with the addition of a potato or two. A villager, with the prospect of just a few plain potatoes for his dinner, obliges, the potatoes are chopped and thrown in the pot. Tasting again she said it needs just a hint of onion, an onion appears and is added to the bubbling cauldron. Some carrots, herbs, a little ham, and pepper come forth from the villagers and finally the peasant woman declares that it is sublime. There is more than enough for everyone and the soup is shared out. The villagers agree that the 'stone soup' is the most delicious they have ever eaten; all take their fill and for the first time in months hunger is defeated. The peasant woman carefully extracts the magical stone and is given a comfortable room for the night by the grateful villagers, before making her way to the next village in the morning.

APPLICATION TO HEALTHCARE

The stone itself possess no magic of course; although it does produce a 'magical' result. The story is an allegory about the power of belief and the inherent ability of a community or team to be able to achieve those things that were previously deemed impossible. The magic was there all along – the community had the elements it needed but it took powerful leadership and a central vision to enable them to work collectively. On their own a few potatoes or a sorry carrot won't make much of a dent in hunger but shared as part of a recipe they can make much more of a difference.

The story of stone soup strikes me as very relevant for the National Health Service (NHS) and other healthcare systems. Incredible improvements in service can be achieved when staff work collectively for the benefit of their patients. Sometimes at the start of the improvement journey, the task can feel hopeless and impossible; the ambition can even seem ridiculous. The role of the leader can be described as creating a vision of the future that is attractive, and demonstrating confidence and determination that this vision is possible, such that others will share this belief.

HOPE

The power of belief in inspiring change is a theme of Helen Bevan's when she writes:

> Hope is the antidote to fear. There is a growing body of evidence about the impact of hopeful actions that every NHS leader should take notice of, particularly in these tough times ... The driving force of hope is belief. As NHS leaders, we have to believe that changes can be made and that we can make them. It is only through our own hopeful thinking (and its demonstration) that we create the capacity to generate and enhance hopeful thinking and action in those we lead.[1]

However, hospitals – my own area of experience for the past 20 years – are strikingly complex places, and at times a phenomenally ambitious goal is needed to simplify what staff are striving for and make success possible. Toward the end of his career, the esteemed management guru Peter Drucker,[2] who had worked across most aspects of the private sector, decided to turn his attention to the US health service and emerged somewhat bewildered, declaring: 'Even small healthcare institutions are complex, barely manageable places ... large healthcare institutions may be the most complex organizations in human history'.[2]

Because of this complexity, achieving change in hospitals can sometimes feel impossible. The message from the stone soup fable is that with a strong enough vision, inspiring belief, the community – in our case staff – can be mobilised to find solutions through working collectively.

SETTING THE AMBITION

As the director of operations in a busy teaching district hospital, the Whittington, in north London, I found setting the ambition to be tremendously important. The NHS can be a real political football, such that the landscape, rules, incentives and systems change with alarming regularity. While it is important for board members to keep up to speed with these changes, it is perhaps just as important to protect staff from them at times, to avoid distracting people with too many unrelated objectives, and to maintain focus on the key big things that make a difference to patients. Often the vision that you ask staff to espouse needs to be relatively long-term, and en route there can be many barriers to achievement, but holding one's nerve and keeping the faith remains very important, as does allowing the team sufficient space and autonomy to achieve the vision their way.

The Whittington's maternity service has a well-deserved excellent reputation and an emphasis on normal birth. We were looking to expand our service and create a birth centre dedicated to midwifery-led care; we decided to be ambitious about this and aim to create the best birth centre in the country. One of the interesting effects of ambitious goals is that they can inspire others and attract them to the work more effectively than modest goals. At an early point we approached Janet Balaskas, the woman who began the 'active birth' movement, whose centre for yoga and birth preparation was by chance just around the corner from the hospital. Janet is an expert, nay guru, on normal birth, and was delighted to be involved in the work to design the best birth centre we possibly could, with features that help support the hormonal response in labour, and a birth pool in every room. Just as in the stone soup allegory, we had within our community the answers to the questions we sought; by starting with an ambitious vision, we gained interest from those best placed to help.

In terms of convincing people to believe that an audacious goal is possible, the view from the top is key, as this sets direction. It is critical that the senior team and, ideally, the trust board believe in what you seek to achieve, and the more ambitious the goal is, the more important it is to have top-team support.

In 2011–12 the maximum threshold for meticillin-resistant *Staphylococcus aureus* bacteraemia at University College London Hospitals NHS Foundation Trust was five. There was considerable scepticism about the achievability of this, and before the start of the year it was highlighted to monitor as a significant risk. The chief nurse, Katherine Fenton, outlined to the executive board that scepticism could be dangerous and could lead to self-fulfilling prophecies. She stated that her belief was that the senior team needed to get behind this and the first step was believing that it was possible and not allowing people to state the impossibility of it but, rather, to use that energy to work on solutions. This we agreed to do and the trust achieved only five bacteraemia that year. 'Hope is an overt choice that we make as leaders',[1] as Bevan says.

'THE CURRENCY OF LEADERSHIP IS ATTENTION'

Dr Jim Reinertsen, a compelling public speaker, is also a former hospital chief executive officer (CEO) and now a leader at the Institute of Healthcare Improvement in Cambridge, Massachusetts Boston, the pre-eminent global improvement centre for healthcare. He uses a phrase that, for me, sums it up beautifully: 'the currency of leadership is attention'.[3] If you care about something, and want others to do so too, and you happen to be in the fortunate position of being a leader, then all you must do is pay attention to that thing and others will watch and do so too. That is your 'currency' as a leader. But sometimes, you will need to pay it an awful lot of attention.

Leaders vary hugely, of course, in their makeup; however, evidence demonstrates that many leaders in the NHS and beyond tend to be at the end of the psychological spectrum that is more active and dynamic – they like to get things done and move onto the next thing. In the language of Belbin: a shaper, rather than a completer finisher.[4] However, sometimes you need to pay an issue a great deal of attention and keep on doing so, even when you might have preferred to move onto the next thing. There is another saying: that you need to communicate a message eight times using eight different media before all staff will have heard it. Essentially, even when you and those around you are entirely bored of reiterating the message, it may still not be out there among front-line teams.

CRACKING 'BARE BELOW THE ELBOW'

If you have ever spent any time on a ward in an NHS hospital, you will have seen groups of young men and women who look identical to new graduates of any profession. Carrying piles of paper and files, smartly turned out, not yet world weary, they could, with a different background, be trainee accountants or lawyers. Only the bleep or a stethoscope reveals them as belonging to one of the clinical professions. Nurses, by contrast, are clearly denoted as such. The seniority nuances within the colours of the uniforms may pass the casual observer by, but in their short-sleeved practical dress or tunic with trousers, and pinned-on watch, it is almost always clear which ones are members of the nursing profession.

At the London hospital where I was chief executive, my director of infection control, May, and I were concerned about infection rates of *Clostridium difficile* in particular; we wanted to make changes that were really significant – if possible, game-changing. One day, at my regular monthly one-to-one with her, we were debating how to crack 'bare below the elbow'. That is, how to ensure that on entering any clinical area all staff removed coats and jackets, hung them up securely, removed watches and any wrist jewellery, and rolled up their sleeves above the elbow in order that they could decontaminate their hands and arms to a sufficient standard of cleanliness.

She suggested to me that we consider providing uniforms for medical staff to ensure we were able to comply with best infection control practice. She and the director of human resources had recently held a session with a group of doctors in training. Medical students undertaking their programme of professional education had asked how they could reduce what they carry onto wards and into departments, and how they could ensure at all times that hand hygiene could be carried out fully. The discussion moved onto secure areas for jackets, coats, handbags, wallets and valuables; this was clearly a real problem for these doctors. The question, 'what would it take to resolve this?' was asked, and I was told that as part of this discussion the suggestion of a uniform emerged from the doctors themselves. They put it that if there were good facilities for showering, changing and storage of property, they would be happy to use these and to change into short-sleeved scrubs or whatever before entering clinical areas.

I thought this was a superb idea; however, there were clearly many dimensions to it. What was gold dust in terms of change management was the fact that the idea had come from the doctors themselves.

However, I didn't think that 'scrubs' would cut it. 'Scrubs' are those loose cotton pyjama-like outfits that are designed for use in hot operating theatres, usually pale green or pale blue. Popular with staff, as they are very comfortable and easy to move in, they are also baggy, with a deeply slashed neckline and made of a washed-out cotton, and I felt that they were not sufficiently presentable or professional. We were looking for something that was a closer equivalent to a suit suitable for medical professionals.

May had looked into this and found another option, newly announced by the manufacturer. This was a short-sleeved tunic top and slimline trousers, available in a dark navy with silver pinstripe, with a large pocket at the front for bleeps, and the word DOCTOR embroidered on the chest. The pinstripe contained real silver and the manufacturer was promoting the fact that silver is naturally antimicrobial. For us this wasn't the point, but here we had an extremely professional-looking proposal. May got hold of some trial uniforms and tested them with the doctors, who liked them.

With the medical director on board, we decided to mandate uniforms for doctors in training from the next intake, and while there were issues – from sizing to ordering to storage in between, I well remember the day when I walked onto a ward and finally saw every single doctor in these fantastic new uniforms. They looked crisp, professional, assured and modern. What was fascinating was how much patients and their relatives liked the uniforms. Above all, they could clearly identify when they had encountered a doctor.

STRATEGIC VERSUS OPERATIONAL FOCUS

Within the literature on leadership, there is much emphasis on the importance of senior leaders, and particularly chief executives, maintaining a strategic focus. The recommendation is often to be ruthless with one's time and to spend it on the key big issues facing the organisation, delegating everything else to members of the team, and certainly not spending time on the minutiae.

It is, of course, critical to keep focus on the wider strategic issues, such as where the organisation is heading, key relationships and how staff and patients in the hospital are feeling. Too often the operational cry of a busy, pressurised healthcare organisation can leave its leaders providing none of this focus.

Stephen Ramsden OBE, an inspirational healthcare leader and early patient safety activist, describes how, when leading a hospital as a CEO, he gradually delegated the operational running of the trust to his executive team. Instead of chairing the weekly operational meeting, he would use the time to get out into the hospital.

'What is the role of a chief executive?' I constantly ask myself this and I firmly believe the NHS has got it wrong. Too much emphasis is placed on operational performance, constantly reinforced by the wider NHS performance management culture. The interpretation of personal accountability often seems to translate into the chief executive signing letters of complaint, and hospital infection data returns, and tracking out-of-network intensive unit transfers.

The symbolism has fostered the wrong emphasis on the chief executive role. Many of us have neglected the really important objective of transforming our organisations, setting ambitious improvement goals (way beyond national targets), being visible to our staff and developing talent in our organisations.

I have begun to change my role dramatically. On the premise that to achieve transformational change you must first change yourself, I have transferred the reporting line for clinical directors from myself to the medical director, and stopped attending weekly executive team meetings.

The changes allow me to spend 30 minutes a day on walkabout. It is the first time in my 16-year chief executive career that I have found a visibility formula that works for me. It has put me back in touch. I feel better, staff feel better and, hopefully, we will change some of the cultural barriers that are so frustrating for all ... I can now spend more time on reducing our hospital standardised mortality rate and patient safety. Nothing should be more important to chief executives than saving lives and showing their staff they care about this ...

Many chief executives are probably already doing all this. But some may still be stuck in an operational role that they feel is warranted by their financial problems. The role of the chief needs to be re-examined. We can be so much more effective than we have been allowed to be.[5]

Stephen used his time to build and maintain strong relationships with his clinical teams, and he witnessed first-hand how patient safety was being considered and how staff and patients were feeling. He was also role-modelling to his leadership team the importance of visibility and in Lean Management terminology, 'going to the gemba' – going to the workplace and seeing for yourself how the service is working. What Stephen tried is admirable and takes real bravery. I believe that if more chief executives were able to lead in this way, we would have a stronger and more effective NHS. As he says, 'If the chief executive is not leading transformational change there is a good chance no one is'.[5]

This is important, as the hospital leadership climate links to the quality of patient care. This has been evidenced by a number of studies including a 2011 report by Michael West[6] and colleagues cited by the NHS Leadership Academy:

Drawing on data from the annual NHS Staff Survey and other sources, the report 'shows how good management of NHS staff leads to higher quality of care, more satisfied patients and lower patient mortality' (2011: 2).

By giving staff clear direction, good support and treating them fairly and supportively, leaders create cultures of engagement, where dedicated NHS staff in turn can give of their best in caring for patients. The analysis of the data shows this can be achieved by focusing on the quality of patient care; ensuring that all staff and their teams have clear objectives; supporting staff via enlightened Human Resource Management practices such as effective appraisal and high quality training; creating positive work climates; building trust and ensuring team working is effective.

The authors say that these elements together can lead to high quality patient care and effective financial performance. Employee engagement is shown to be especially important. This in turn is seen as fostered by effective leadership and management. A number of correlations were revealed with staff engagement 'having significant associations with patient satisfaction, patient mortality, infection rates, Annual Health Check scores, as well as staff absenteeism and turnover. The more engaged staff members are, the better the outcomes for patients and the organisation generally'.

ROLE OF THE SPONSOR: ENSURING DELIVERY

However, having said that, it is important to note that sometimes the minutiae really matter. Within every key campaign will be an element of detail, which, if disregarded, could stall the whole change. When senior leaders sponsor work, they need to find this problem and solve it, regardless of the level of detail involved.

There were numerous examples of this within the uniform campaign; obtaining lockers, building shower and changing facilities, sorting out padlocks, for instance. However, the one that really stays with me is that it was only as we took delivery of uniforms, just before go-live, that it became apparent that the trousers arrived un-hemmed.

There was a school of thought that the uniforms could be given out like this, with doctors in training responsible for hemming the trousers. My view was that this was impractical, and if we were serious about giving this the best chance of success we needed to make it error-proof – that is, as straightforward as possible for our doctors to comply with the new system.

The manager of the education centre had been put in charge of the project, which was a good move, as she had the right approach, being bright and motivated to succeed, and she was also in a useful position in the organisation, as building strong relationships with doctors in training was part of her role.

The consultant medical staff at that trust were in the habit of taking lunch together in the education centre, and I used to join them, typically twice a week, to catch up informally. It was a great way of getting into conversation with a good range of consultants, to understand the mood of the organisation, and it was almost always very entertaining.

As the project took off, I would call in to the manager during these visits, to check on progress and see if all was going well. At one of these sessions she suggested that a member of her team who had dressmaking skills could do fittings with each of the doctors and then hem the trousers correctly over a number of evenings; this way we could quickly get the issue sorted. I endorsed this and made arrangements for the individual to be paid overtime for her needlework. Now the leadership gurus would no doubt be tutting at me wildly by this point, for getting so involved in the operational detail rather than maintaining a strategic focus, but I see this issue as critical and in so many projects a great idea fails to launch 'for want of a nail'.

Without this type of consideration, delivery of the goal would have been affected. Attention to details as microscopic as these is required to ensure a successful campaign, and, as Reinertsen points out, this attention is the very currency of leadership.

A Department of Health visit that took place after the introduction of uniforms for medical staff stated that we were the best hospital that they had visited across the NHS in terms of our compliance with 'bare below the elbow'.

COURAGE AND COMMITMENT

Leaders also need to demonstrate personal courage and commitment if we are to constantly innovate in our approach to these key safety issues. Another area that needs to be addressed when tacking *C. difficile* is the use of antimicrobials. Reducing the availability of broad-spectrum antibiotics is now a clearly understood and evidenced part of the reduction of rates of *C. difficile*. However, in 2007 it was a rather different story. As part of our work, we invited in the Department of Health expert Professor Brian Duerden to review all aspects of our infection control work and to help us draw up our microbial policy. He did so and we implemented it.

However, there was considerable resistance and opposition, which claimed that we had gone too far in our antimicrobial policy – further, it was argued, than any other trust in the NHS was going at that time – that patients would be at risk as we miss infections, that length of stay would undoubtedly increase, particularly in our extremely efficient acute medicine unit, which would create serious flow issues within the hospital. All this from well-respected consultants, including those expert in clinical pharmacology, which made for some difficult medical committees.

Some of the opposition seemed to be about more than the issue at hand; perhaps the change was more profound than we had appreciated. Atul Gawande, is a surgeon and Harvard academic who has written very compellingly on the negative impact of medical hierarchy on surgical safety, in his excellent books *Better* and *The Checklist Manifesto*. In a BBC interview on the impact of the surgical checklist, he says: 'There's tremendous hierarchy in an operating room, and when people get a chance to say their name out loud, it actually changes the likelihood that they will speak up later when they have a problem or have any doubts',[7] and the surgical safety checklist has been described as a tool to help flatten hierarchy and thereby increase safety.

I don't think it is unreasonable to suppose that hierarchies exist across medicine, albeit in the minds of some rather than in reality, and I believe that what may have been at the bottom of the fierceness of the opposition was that 'backroom' clinicians such as microbiologists were restricting the clinical autonomy of 'field' doctors. People could no longer prescribe as they had done, and the truth was that we didn't fully know what the implications of this would be.

Before one medical committee I suggested to May, who is petite, that as I happened to have a custom-made size 8 flak jacket in my loft (belonging to a dear friend who was then a war correspondent), I should bring it in for her to wear at the next meeting as a visual prop. We toughed this out together, the medical director met with those who behaved inappropriately, but even so it was very demanding to lead for infection control at this time.

The policy was agreed and implemented and we monitored performance closely, bringing it back to key meetings such as the board of directors, hospital management board and the medical committee.

COMMUNICATING THE CHANGE

The Institute for Healthcare Improvement run a fantastic conference on executive leadership and safety, reputed to be the best globally. I was fortunate enough to be sponsored to attend by the NHS Institute for Innovation and Improvement when working with them on developing the Productive Operating Theatre. Within this programme the role of executive leadership is identified as being to provide direction and to build in a way that will make the past become unacceptable and the future appear more attractive. In doing this, particularly explaining why the status quo won't do and why alternatives are desirable, as well as necessary, communications play a major role.

At the trust where I was working, the communications function had been outsourced. The aim had been to raise the profile of communications including external coverage, and a firm had been selected that had good political insight, which was seen as a distinct advantage. These aims are, of course, laudable and the outsourced provider did a good job in these areas. However, my very strong feeling was that the trust needed to focus much more strongly on its internal communications and that it was always going to be very difficult for an outside agency based in central London, where clients were almost exclusively private sector, to achieve the intimacy required to pull off great internal communications in a trust near Twickenham.

So on my recommendation the board took the decision to end the contract and rebuild the in-house team. Considerable revamping then took place of the trust's newspaper, the website and other media, and we were one of the first hospitals to use film as a medium for patients to learn more about our facilities.

We made these changes to our communications setup because we felt that to build our reputation further we needed to start with the messages to our own staff. While the changes weren't directly linked to the infection control work, having a switched on, responsive and energetic in-house communications team was key to launching effective infection control campaigns.

THE IMPACT

And the rates? They plummeted. *C. difficile* is a truly horrible disease. It is extremely painful, it is debilitating, it takes away dignity and, indeed, it can take away life. If you contract *C. difficile* or – more provocatively but not unfairly so – if we give you it, your chances of dying are increased. The mortality rate looks from studies to be 6%–30%.[8]

The differences in our rates between the first quarter of 2007 to the second was a drop of 40%. Had the first-quarter rate continued, we would have been looking at 316 cases that year; instead, we had 178, and in the following year this was down to 123. Rates per 100 000 bed days reduced from 140.4 to 94.8.[9] There was plenty more to do to get them down further – every case is one too many – but it seemed that control had been gained and those very high historic rates have never been returned to.

The data demonstrate a reduction in the rate of *C. difficile* at the hospital after implementing this wide range of measures. It is hard to attribute benefits to particular schemes but clearly the overall impact was positive. The improvement has continued for subsequent quarters and not returned to the pre-2008 levels. It should be noted that when looking at the performance data in retrospect, the first quarter of 2007 was a particularly high period for *C. difficile* for the trust (regardless of location of origin being community or hospital-acquired), with a number of prior quarters and years being considerably lower.

APPROACHES TO MEETING THE QUALITY AND EFFICIENCY CHALLENGE

Surviving the most significant and sustained period of financial constraint in NHS history while retaining the quality has been called 'the biggest challenge facing the NHS' by its then chief executive, Sir David Nicholson, in 2009.[10] This was reiterated in 2014 by his replacement as incoming CEO of NHS England, Simon Stevens, when he said:

> we meet ... at a defining moment in the history of our National Health Service. A time when the standards of care for the vast majority of our communities continues to be extremely high ... but also a time of the most intense public focus ever on the quality and safety and dignity of our care ... Coinciding with the most sustained budget crunch since the Second World War. Now in Year Five of essentially flat health funding.[11]

University College London NHS Foundation Trust (UCLH) is a large central London trust made up of seven hospitals. It is a busy trust, providing a range of local and more specialist services and undertaking a large research portfolio. UCLH is also part of UCL Partners, the world's largest academic health science system. An early foundation trust, UCLH did very well out of the years of growth, successfully growing its national and local services in line with the investment in health services that was made by the Blair and Brown administrations.

With the global economic recession, increases to NHS budgets ceased, and this combined with rising demand led to significant challenges. UCLH began its work on meeting the quality and efficiency challenge in January 2010. As lead director, I established a small programme office and launched the trust's approach to Quality, Efficiency and Productivity (QEP).

The aim was to make sustained financial savings, while maintaining the hard-won quality gains for which we were known – such as being rated among the best hospitals in London for patient experience and having one of the best survival rates in the country.

The UCLH QEP programme established a number of principles.

- *Involvement of Everyone*: part of core work, led by operational leaders, all staff involved, strong communications element

- *Make Life Simple*: using Lean as our method, simplifying processes wherever possible
- *Keep Patients Safe*: the mantra that safer care is cheaper; minimise harm, including falls, infections, pressure ulcers
- *Use the Evidence*: be better at learning from elsewhere, events and visits programme
- *Spend Money Wisely*: ensure that every purchasing decision is as good as it can be.

Using information for improvement was seen as central from the start and the key performance metrics, which include quality, efficiency and productivity measures, are all presented as statistical process control charts. Because statistical process control charts demonstrate real shifts rather than normal variation, they are well suited for documenting changes linked to improvement work.

UCLH has a highly devolved, clinically led structure and the QEP programme is based on this. The vast majority of schemes are implemented at a local level and overseen by the relevant medical director and clinical board. The programme office focuses on supporting change in trust-wide schemes and also coordinates reporting on progress. In its first 4 years, the programme has achieved recurrent efficiency savings of over £140 million, with quality markers continuing to improve.

Returning to the analogy that opened this chapter, the QEP programme has had plenty of 'stone soup' moments. A reduction in spend on agency staff of 75% has been achieved through a vision of working entirely without agency staff, using our own staff or those on our staff bank, who know the trust well. The first department to achieve this was the busy maternity service, who got to zero agency midwives, a real triumph in a service where continuity is so important but frequently eludes us. It is heartening to see that the power of belief, underpinned by excellent process change, and clinicians and managers working together for patients, can deliver a level of change that could perhaps be described as miraculous.

REFERENCES

1. Bevan H. Who's afraid of the big bad wolf? *Health Serv J.* 2011; **121**(6239): 14–15.
2. Drucker P. *Managing in the Next Society.* New York: Truman Talley Books; 2002.
3. Reinertson JL, Pugh M, Bisognano M. *Seven Leadership Leverage Points for Organization-level improvement in health care.* Cambridge, MA: Institute for Healthcare Improvement; 2005.
4. Belbin M (1981). *Management Teams: why they succeed or fail.* Heinemann ISBN 0-470-27172-8.
5. Ramsden S. On being a good chief executive. *Health Serv J.* 2007; **117**(6073): 34.

6. West M, Dawson J, Admasachew L, *et al. NHS Staff Management and Health Service Quality: results from the NHS Staff Survey and related data.* London: Department of Health; 2011. Available at: www.gov.uk/government/publications/nhs-staff-management-and-health-service-quality (accessed 23 June 2015).

7. Lee D. *Dr Atul Gawande's Checklist for Saving Lives.* BBC World Service; 2010 Feb 5.

8. Hota S, Achonu C, Crowcroft N, *et al.* Determining mortality rates attributable to *Clostridium difficile* infection. *Emerg Infect Dis J.* 2012; **18**(2): 305–7.

9. *Clostridium difficile*: updated guidance on diagnosis and reporting. Department of Health. www.gov.uk/government/publications/updated-guidance-on-the-diagnosis-and-reporting-of-clostridium-difficile

10. Nicholson D. *The Year: NHS Chief Executive's annual report 2008/09.* London: Department of Health; 2009. www.gov.uk/government/publications/department-of-health-departmental-report-2009 (accessed 24 June 2015).

11. Stevens S. Thinking like a patient, acting like a taxpayer – from NHS challenges to new solutions? Speech at NHS Confederation Annual Conference, 2014 June 4. Liverpool www.england.nhs.uk/2014/06/04/simon-stevens-speech-confed/

CHAPTER 4

Infection prevention and control in the operating department: a student's perspective

....

Taraneh Azizi

Operating Department Practitioners (ODPs) and theatre personnel have direct involvement in infection control issues,[1] as it is a part of their everyday working practice. Student ODPs are constantly reminded of the importance of infection control during their pre-registration training.[2] There is distinct and continued dedication within this area in the academic institutions that provide the relevant healthcare programmes. Infection prevention and control plays a large part in the ODP programme but applies to all staff members who work in theatres, which is not limited to ODPs but also comprises registered and non-registered staff. Surgical site infections are one of the many types of healthcare-associated infections (HCAIs) that patients are at risk of contracting following a visit to the operating department, as patients are at higher risk and are more vulnerable than usual because of the nature of such invasive procedures being carried out.[3]

> Write down a list of five activities in your clinical practice that are relevant to infection prevention and control, and give an example in each activity of what would be considered suboptimal practice.

Healthcare students based in the operating department are given a broad exposure to the implications of substandard infection control. Examples include provision of statistics relating to HCAIs, the aetiology of infections, the different types of infection, and preventive methods used in the healthcare environment. The theatre environment has more considerations than simply undertaking hand hygiene; there are many wider issues associated with infection control in the operating department, including surgical hand asepsis, prepping and draping, gowning and gloving, and instrument decontamination.[4]

As part of the professional education and clinical training given, student ODPs are made fully aware of the importance of infection control and surrounding issues. These include fundamental issues such as personal hygiene, and suitable attire being worn in and around the theatre environment. In all clinical areas, there should at least be personal protective equipment (PPE) available such as eye protection and disposable gloves and aprons at a minimum.[5] However, there are also more complex issues, such as what is considered sterile and unsterile, and within the sterile area what is considered to be 'clean' and 'dirty'. These are included in a variety of modules within healthcare programmes to reiterate the application of infection control and represent them in different areas within their work setting. Therefore, students can identify the application of infection prevention and control within a variety of areas aimed at demonstrating best practice that is evidence based.[6]

Students are given the most current and up-to-date research supported through healthcare journals and other academic reading material. Infection control is a pertinent issue in the operating department, as there are severe implications when infection prevention methods are not followed or best practice is not demonstrated. Patients who are exposed to a surgical environment are at risk of infection from the surgery alone, irrespective of the complexity of surgery being undertaken. Part of the 'chain of infection' means that infection can be introduced through various routes in this environment: invasive monitoring, non-sterile contact, poor ventilation and instrument contamination.[7] Where potential routes of infection are controlled and prevented, the highest possible standard of care can be delivered and patients experience safer surgery.[8] Students receive training at taught sessions at their academic institutions, but they also receive training on placements from existing staff within theatres.[9]

Typical daily infection control considerations for the ODP would begin before the practitioner even enters the department. The practitioner must ensure that he or she has demonstrated high standards of personal hygiene and washed his or her hands before entering the theatre suite. Suitable theatre blues and theatre shoes provided by the department must be worn, and these are not removed from the department.[10] In addition, theatre attire is washed at certain temperatures by linen services for the hospital. All jewellery must be removed, with the exception of simple stud earrings or a plain wedding band. Hair must be tied up and covered with a disposable theatre hat, provided by the department. The theatre practitioner can then enter the operating suite and begin the working day.[11]

Daily tasks include scrubbing up for surgical procedures, whereby surgical hand asepsis is carried out before every operation by all staff in the sterile area immediately around the operation site. The first scrub of the day is performed with a nail brush. Scrubbing up needs to be with a suitable scrub solution and following the appropriate standards for surgical scrub technique.[12] The practitioner will then gown and glove and approach his or her instrument set, which contains sterile surgical instrumentation and supplementary swabs, sharps and other countable items. Some patients may need shaving immediately prior to surgery and selection of a suitable prep solution for the skin will be required. The theatre practitioner will assist the surgeon by passing instruments within the sterile area and ensuring the sterility of the equipment being used during surgery and accounting for all instruments, sharps and items used during each operation.[13]

At the end of the procedure, all items and instruments are accounted for and all gowns, gloves and waste from the operation goes into the appropriate clinical waste bag and is removed from the theatre into the 'dirty' or sluice corridor.[14] The theatre practitioner then has to clean the theatre before the next patient arrives and, after all cleaning is completed, hand washing is exercised by all theatre staff before contact with the next patient. This is repeated depending on the number of cases in each theatre, but theatres may need time to 'stand' or equipment may need to be removed from the theatre before certain known infected cases.

Each task actually has vast implications for infection control and should be considered in what is best practice. For example, a part of everyday theatre practice is scrubbing for surgery. It is not as simple as routine hand washing. Hands must be kept higher than elbows at all times to ensure that 'dirty' solution or water runs down the arms and not onto 'clean' hands. Rinsing must take place in this same position for the same reasons. The six-step scrub procedure must be followed to ensure that all areas of the hands are washed with scrub solution. Even drying of the hands must be done in a certain way; using the opposite hand to dry the other hand, starting from the hand and working down to the elbow and vice versa on the other hand with a separate sterile paper towel. Theatre practitioners must always be aware of where they are and what they are doing, to ensure they are demonstrating best practice in relation to infection prevention and control. As a student, this is a lot of information to take on board in the theatre environment. All of a sudden, there are things you cannot touch or be near because you are considered 'unsterile'. This is quite different from any other healthcare environment.

There are a lot of considerations for the theatre practitioner when working in an operating department. The manner in which sterile supplementaries are opened, the way that practitioners gown and glove up prior to surgery and many other daily theatre activities must be carefully considered, to ensure that infection prevention and control standards are appropriately met.[5] This is crucial because surgical site infections are one of the biggest groups of infections acquired in the healthcare environment.

Infection control and prevention is a remarkable area in healthcare. Numerous colleagues and staff members are able to identify times where they have witnessed poor practice in relation to infection control, and unfortunately these matters often go unchallenged. Students and newly qualified staff are generally not in a position to challenge practice that comes from staff more senior to them. Students, in particular, are faced with the continual challenge of engaging in poor practice because mentors request that the practice of their students should echo their own. Students can perceive negative attitudes toward infection prevention and control from qualified practitioners, and this can impede student learning. This should be the opportunity to eliminate poor infection control from the operating department and set the standard for a better future. Mentors should work toward overcoming barriers to good infection prevention practice.[15]

From personal experience, I found during my programme of professional education that students were arriving at and undertaking clinical placements with a different level of knowledge than some of their mentors. In fact, and as controversial as it may sound, the knowledge and practice of some students is far superior to that of their seniors.[16] Thus it is important to recognise that learning is and always will be a two way process where students and their mentors can learn from each other.

For example, personal experience yielded a situation where a theatre practitioner attempted to demonstrate surgical hand asepsis through scrubbing prior to surgery. The practitioner was considered a senior member of staff because of the longevity of the practitioner's service, and resulting experience in a variety of areas. The scrub-up process that the theatre practitioner demonstrated as current practice (and practice therefore that the theatre practitioner is teaching to students) had since been superseded by newer and more current techniques. The demonstration included a scrub time of 5–10 minutes with a surgical scrub solution in at least three different scrubs. The first scrub was up to and including the elbows, the second scrub was just below the elbows and the third scrub included the hands and wrists only. Current guidelines[11] state that two scrubs of 2 minutes' minimum time with an appropriate antiseptic solution is a suitable scrub procedure prior to surgery. Although it is not poor practice to scrub for longer than this, new evidence has suggested that there is no added benefit by scrubbing for longer than 2 minutes.[17]

The extent to which some registered staff are unaware of current standards or guidelines regarding infection control is concerning for the students who are mentored by them. This also has implications for patients where they witness staff perhaps not carrying out hand washing where they feel the staff should. Patients reflect positively towards healthcare professionals who are visibly seen to take precautions on hand washing during their care. The practitioner who demonstrated the dated practice as described earlier is not alone. Infection control awareness extends to a range of practitioners who work within the operating department. For example, surgeons have been seen to use alcohol scrub as their first scrub of the day, and hands are often seen to not be kept higher than the elbows as part of their scrub technique.[18] Similarly, anaesthetists have been seen to not scrub or gown up prior to a spinal anaesthetic; scrubbing up for a spinal anaesthetic is a crucial part of best practice during this type of anaesthetic because of the invasive nature of the procedure. Healthcare assistants have also been seen to not wear hats in the necessary clinical areas; the list goes on.

There is a strong element of ritualistic behaviour in localised environments. Despite ongoing work and more current research around evidenced-based practice relating to more up-to-date clinical practices, elements of nursing remain traditional. Clinical judgement is being undermined, while routines and rituals seem to be guiding care pathways. This in effect limits the possibility of positive change.[19] Although the issues here are quite complex and change is progressive, the sense of security that rituals provide overrides practice in clinical areas because of the sense of security that rituals and traditions provide to nursing staff.

> Consider a student practitioner of a different discipline within health and social care. Give an example of an additional issue regarding infection prevention and control that you think affects the student in his or her particular specialty.

From a student perspective, it is disappointing to have experiences in clinical practice that are so different to what is being taught at university. The conflicting teachings are inconsistent with one another, and it can be confusing and challenging for students to accept what, in fact, is best practice. Students need more consistency and clarity with infection control. All staff who work in theatres need a much stricter and better-defined record of continuing professional development that will document competency and knowledge relating to infection control in their work environment on a regular basis. The e-learning systems that are currently available are not an effective method of recording regular updates.[20]

In an alternative placement, personal experience has identified other infection prevention and control issues that are equally important, outside of the operating department. In a ward setting across an emergency care centre and a clinical decision unit, the practice of practitioners is much more open and practice feels, to an extent, under continual scrutiny. This appears in the form of relatives, colleagues and infection control link nurses. Personally, it was evident that this feeling of being watched made the practitioner more aware of their practice and particularly at times when the practitioner was in the presence of others.

In the ward environment, the student practitioner is introduced to an environment that is very different to the familiarity of an operating theatre. The concern of strict surgical asepsis and sterility is diminished, and replaced by the seemingly basic tasks of everyday ward nursing. This includes changing bed linen, assistance with personal care and use of commodes. As a student, the change in environment was incredibly challenging from an infection prevention and control perspective.

There was an incident where an infection prevention and control link nurse performed a routine inspection on the ward that resulted in the student practitioner being identified as demonstrating incorrect infection control practice. The task being performed was a bed linen change, a task that distressed a patient due to pain on movement. Therefore, the bed linen had to be changed with the patient still on the bed, and this was achieved by the patient rolling from side to side while the linen was changed by two attending practitioners: the student and a healthcare assistant. The patient was calling out in pain during the process, and so the bed was changed quickly to avoid further distress to the patient. When the bed was changed and cleaned down with sanitising wipes, the student practitioner then took the linen from the patient's bedside over to the nearest red laundry sack. The infection control link nurse witnessed this action and pulled the student to one side, explaining that this was not the correct way to have performed that particular task. It was explained to the student practitioner that to avoid spreading potential infection, any used bed linen is considered as soiled, and therefore a suitable laundry sack should be moved to the patient's bedside, rather than transferring dirty linen across the ward to the laundry sack.

It was not that the student practitioner was not aware of how to perform this task to the accepted standard; rather, the priority for the student at that time had been to minimise the distress to the patient, and infection prevention and control was potentially compromised by this action. This is an example of how a fundamental task performed on a daily basis can have implications for infection prevention and control. In this instance, the student practitioner had followed what other qualified staff on the ward had been doing, and this shows how important the student/mentor learning relationship can be in influencing infection prevention and control in the future. It can be confusing for students who are trying to balance what they have been taught at university with what they are told to do in practice; often there is a conflict between the two, which should not be occurring in modern-day practice.

Infection control is a practical part of everyday practice that is clearly not being adhered to and prevention is a core element of patient safety. Monitoring of continuing professional development is essential in providing safer healthcare practices.[21]

> Your mentor demonstrates to you how to perform hand hygiene and then asks you to copy the practice. The hand hygiene that your mentor demonstrates is not what you believe to be in line with local policy and the evidence-based practice you have been taught on your course. What do you do?

SUMMARY

Student healthcare practitioners should be taught the most current and highest standards of infection control practice, relating to evidence-based practice supported by a number of academic resources. This requirement is often inconsistent with the experiences of students on clinical placement, and this has the potential to affect the future practice of these students as registered healthcare practitioners. Ultimately, this affects patient care, treatment and outcome. Students can be exposed to poor practice on a regular basis and so need more support from senior staff, especially when presented with conflicting practices from mentors. Teaching staff thus need to ensure that they are current and up to date with evidence-based practice and guidelines that are in line with the academic content from the student's university or college. Hospital trusts need to review infection control training and competency of their staff to ensure that patient safety is not compromised.

> Taraneh Azizi has now been qualified for 2 years and is working as a registered ODP in the main theatre department at the Royal United Hospital in Bath.

REFERENCES

1. Williams M. Infection control and prevention in perioperative practice. *J Perioper Pract.* 2008; **18**(7): 274–8.
2. Harvey P. Role of the mentor in the theatre setting. *J Perioper Pract.* 2012; **22**(7): 232–6.
3. Wilson R. Minimising the spread of infection in the operating department. *J Perioper Pract.* 2012; **22**(6): 185–8.
4. Wilson J, Loveday H, Hoffman P, *et al.* Uniform: an evidence review of the microbiological significance of uniforms and uniform policy in the prevention and control of healthcare-associated infections. Report to Department of Health (England). *J Hosp Infect.* 2007; **66**(4): 301–7.
5. Pratt R, Pellowe C, Wilson J. National evidence based guidelines for preventing healthcare associated infections in NHS hospitals in England. *J Hosp Infect.* 2007; **65**(Suppl. 1): S1–64.
6. Gopee N. *Mentoring and Supervision in Healthcare.* London: Sage; 2008.
7. Damani N. *Manual of Infection Control Procedures.* 2nd ed. Cambridge: Cambridge University Press; 2003.
8. Al-Benna S. Infection control in operating theatres. *J Perioper Pract.* 2012; **22**(10): 318–22.
9. Richmond S. Minimising the risk of infection in the operating department: a review for practice. *J Perioper Pract.* 2009; **19**(4): 142–6.
10. Sivanandan I, Bowker K, Bannister G, *et al.* Reducing the risk of surgical site infection. *J Perioper Pract.* 2011; **21**(2): 69–72.
11. Association for Perioperative Practice (AfPP) *Standards and Recommendations for Practice.* Harrogate: AfPP; 2011.
12. Dougherty L, Lister S, editors. *The Royal Marsden Hospital Manual of Clinical Nursing Procedures.* Oxford: Wiley-Blackwell; 2011.
13. Wicker P, O'Neill J, editors. *Caring for the Perioperative Patient.* 2nd ed. Oxford: Wiley-Blackwell; 2010.
14. Department of Health. *Health Technical Memorandum 07-01: safe management of healthcare waste.* London: Department of Health; 2006.
15. Ward D. Attitudes towards infection prevention and control. *BMJ Qual Saf.* 2012; **21**(4): 301–6.
16. Azizi T. Young person advisor to the AfPP board. *AfPP Newsletter.* September 2012.
17. Weaving P, Cox F, Milton S. Infection prevention and control in the operating theatre: reducing the risk of surgical site infections (SSIs). *J Perioper Pract.* 2008; **18**(5): 199–204.
18. Pirie S. Hand washing and surgical hand asepsis. *J Perioper Pract.* 2010; **20**(5): 169–72.
19. Zeitz K, McCutcheon H. Traditions, rituals and standards, in a realm of evidence based nursing care. *Contemp Nurse.* 2005; **18**(3): 300–8. Available at: www.contemporarynurse.com/archives/vol/18/issue/3/article/2101/tradition-rituals-and-standards-in-a-realm-of (accessed 13 September 2013).
20. Drayton S. *The Advantages and Disadvantages of eLearning* [blog]. BusinessZone; 13 August 2013. Available at: www.businesszone.co.uk/blogs/scott-drayton/optimus-sourcing/advantages-and-disadvantages-elearning (accessed 23 September 2013).
21. Association for Perioperative Practice (AfPP). *Foundations in Practice.* Harrogate: AfPP; 2010.

CHAPTER 5

The lament

....

Harley Farmer

The nightingale's beautiful song is sung because life isn't going to plan for the bird, despite its best efforts. The song we cherish is a voice of anguish, a lament. It's a message to others of its kind, yet singing at night exposes the nightingale to attack by predators. The message is fine but when it helps predators, the outcome can be problematic. Healthcare professionals, including infection control professionals (ICPs), use peer-reviewed journals to convey their desire to improve outcomes for patients. The message is fine but when it helps antagonistic lawyers, the outcome can be problematic. Is there a useful analogy between the nightingale's song and the healthcare-associated infection (HCAI) profession's literature when both generate exposure to threat? I believe so. The nightingale is not going to change, so it will remain exposed. Change is something the HCAI profession has to use with due caution, as change can bring new dangers. In this chapter, I will suggest failure to change presents a greater danger than change. For years ICPs and others have developed new approaches and products to break HCAI cycles. Regrettably, the 'system' prevents us from fully achieving the aims. Despite our best efforts, many people still die from HCAIs, leaving ICPs with a need to explain why. My novel *The Reaper's Rainbow*[1] takes an understanding of HCAI cycles to the public. Questions woven into the plot bring readers to the realisation that they can play their part in protecting themselves from infections. For a long time they've been told to 'wash your hands' but few do it. The novel delivers a new perspective, allowing them to realise the advantages of change. I favour asking questions, as questions deliver answers. Without the right questions, the right answers remain hidden. Sometimes the right questions can be challenging, and those in this chapter are offered to ICPs in that light.

It can help to view intractable problems such as HCAIs from a different perspective. Using simple psychology tools such as reframing and strategic visioning, I ask people to visualise HCAIs as being very rare. Rather than hoping the deaths could be reduced by even 50%, which would still leave thousands of deaths every year, what if we started at zero and concentrated our efforts on the few that would inevitably happen? The commonest question this induces is: *how*? It's a good question that reliably exposes boundaries and limiting beliefs. I ask you to rearrange the letters in *how* to make *who*. Throughout this chapter, whenever you want to ask *how*? try, instead, asking *who*? *How* tends to highlight barriers, while *who* usually increases resources.

REFLECTION EXERCISE 1

Give yourself a moment to consider those times when you knew what could be done to improve patient safety but you found you had too few resources to take the positive action. How different would things be now if you'd had those resources then?

Considerable progress is being made in infection prevention with the introduction of internationally accepted best practices. There are too many to mention here, so by way of example I will place emphasis on the use of hand rubs. ICPs justifiably point to successes such as meticillin-resistant *Staphylococcus aureus* (MRSA) infections now being less prevalent in Britain than infections due to meticillin-susceptible *S. aureus* (MSSA). Congratulations are due, when viewing from the technical perspective of ICPs. Now consider how it looks from the viewpoint of a family bereaved by an MSSA infection. Changing R to S and congratulating ourselves matters little to them: their loved one is dead. Do we attempt to point out how much better it is that their loved one died from an antibiotic-susceptible bacterium because we've achieved pleasing success against the antibiotic-resistant equivalent? No. We quietly lament in the knowledge that MSSA is a natural part of normal skin flora and predates the introduction of antibiotics. It has always been a potential pathogen, even though the introduction of antibiotics brought MRSA into greater prominence. Did patients who have died from HCAIs enter the hospital with the expectation of only being protected against MRSA? No, they rightly expected to be protected against infection from all pathogens.

DEBATES

There are three simultaneous but distinct debates occurring. ICPs can feel buoyant in the *technical* debate. However, we are judged in the *outcome* debate when people continue to die from infections. It's easier for the public to remember the person who went into hospital for a toe operation and died from infection than it is for them to remember our lengthy proclamations on best practices. In the *outcome* debate, you may well hear the question, 'How *bad* are these *best* practices?' The enormous cost of HCAIs mean the *financial* debate is also disconcerting. Those three debates – technical, outcome and financial – are ongoing.

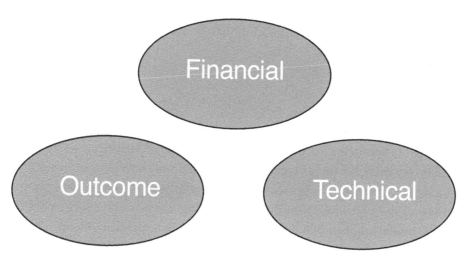

FIGURE 5.1 Three simultaneous but distinct debates

When most emphasis is placed on the *technical* debate, less attention is given to the *outcome* and *financial* debates. In actively partaking in all three debates, I've heard some interesting questions and have raised more of my own, including those presented here. The answers to those questions suggest a lot more can be done to avoid HCAIs. The references cited in this chapter justify that statement. There are complicating factors such as poor adherence to practices and anionic cleansing products chemically inactivating cationic antimicrobial products. If those known weaknesses are inherent in our best practices, can those practices really be deemed entirely fit for purpose? The many peer-reviewed articles highlighting areas where improvements can be made suggest not. Was a family bereaved by an avoidable HCAI best served by current best practices? No.

REFLECTION EXERCISE 2

Take some time to examine the ingredients in the cleansing and antimicrobial products used in your facility. Pay particular attention to whether anionic (negatively charged) and cationic (positively charged) ingredients are ever likely to be used on the same surface, providing the chance to inactivate each other.

Most HCAI discussions focus on the *technical* debate. That would seem reasonable, as it's essential to know whether a product kills pathogens. In the *outcome* debate, people assume the products can kill microbes and ask why those microbes are still killing people? In the *technical* debate the focus is on microbes dying; in the *outcome* debate it's on people dying.

CONFLICT

Wouldn't you agree those two debates appear to be opposites and it would be helpful to reduce the conflict? If so, an obvious question is *how*? That has always revealed barriers. Try *who*? Are there people wanting to help, who haven't been engaged yet? Yes, millions of them. They're the public, especially those who've become patients. It's the patients who develop the infections, perhaps introducing a perspective that patients are the problem. Would it be useful to turn that problem into the solution? Do patients have spare time, do they bring a collective wealth of experience and do they have a personal interest in avoiding lethal infections? Yes; and they don't require payment! Half the people in most hospitals are patients – a massive, largely untapped, human resource.

Another large group in hospitals is healthcare workers. They must be paid, making them an expensive resource. Does it make sense to look after them as best we can? Yes, but does that happen with current best practices? Let's explore one example. Imagine if alcohol hand rubs had never been introduced. What would happen if, in these times of valid health and safety considerations, someone suggested the hands of staff should be doused in a flammable solvent numerous times every day? Laws would prevent any employer introducing such hazardous technology. Yet that is one of the actions that best practices advocate. If it's so wrong, why is it done?

A *technical* answer is that alcohol on hands kills superficial transient bacteria. One counterargument from the *outcome* debate is to ask whether alcohol hand rubs were a major part of the infection prevention strategy throughout the global MRSA epidemic? Could it be that alcohol hand rubs are not stopping lethal bacterial infections? Are numerous lethal bacterial infections happening while alcohol hand rubs are readily available? Arguably, yes is the answer to all three questions. Nobody knows how many patients have been saved by alcohol hand rubs, but evidence from hospitals around the world shows how many patients died from bacterial infections while alcohol hand rubs were at their bedsides. Obviously, alcohol hand rubs are only one component of an overall infection prevention strategy, but if one component that is given such prominence can be challenged so easily, the whole system becomes open to challenge.

Evidence-based research is the basis of best practices, yet any HCAI death suggests evidence of failure to protect that specific patient. ICPs who advocate alcohol hand rubs can counter by saying that the problem lies with staff not using the rubs. That's a valid *technical* riposte, so let's investigate this poor compliance. Chronic hand eczema (product-related dermatitis on the hands) is well known among healthcare workers.[2] Is it reasonable to expect a person with hand dermatitis to apply a flammable solvent to their damaged hands? No. Is there evidence-based research of poor user compliance rates of alcohol hand rub usage? Yes.[3] Yet, we fail to care for those damaged hands when we give alcohol hand rubs great priority in best practices to prevent HCAIs. On this basis, is the term 'best practices' looking more like the 'best *of current* practices'?

REFLECTION EXERCISE 3

What is the incidence of chronic hand eczema (product-related dermatitis on the hands) among the healthcare workers in your facility? Is special provision allowed for them to use effective non-alcohol hand rubs that are deemed to be non-hazardous by your occupational health team? If so, why can't the non-hazardous rub be used by everyone in the facility?

THE ATTACKERS

Now for the *really* challenging questions … the attacker will be a lawyer whose questions may be biased toward unreasonable answers because the lawyer is more interested in a specific legal outcome than any technical niceties. Is all this evidence-based research freely available to lawyers acting against hospitals in cases of lethal HCAIs? Is it reasonable to assume a lawyer could convince a jury that all this evidence was known by the ICP who advocated the use of alcohol hand rubs in the hospital where the HCAI victim died? Could it be argued that the ICP knew there was poor user compliance of the alcohol hand rub and that might have played a part in the failure to save this victim's life? Despite that, did the hospital's ICP still advocated its use? Yes, answers to questions like that favour attack. Some of those questions are undoubtedly unfair from the ICP's *technical* perspective, but the lawyer's aim is to influence the jury of a poor *outcome* from the deceased patient's perspective. This will not be a balanced debate; fairness should not be anticipated.

The nightingale's lament exposes the bird to attack by predators. Researchers and those working for healthcare providers assiduously present their evidence-based research to the world, embellished with their anguish. Their data, their lament, shows that many patients continue to die from HCAIs. Lawyers are poised to attack and anyone who relies on a 'best practice' defence exposes themselves.

Evidence-based research in peer-reviewed journals in the medical, health and social care literature is the basis on which best practices are based. That provides comfort and support from the *technical* viewpoint. It shows we know our current limitations. Now let me demonstrate how easily that same literature can assist aggressive lawyers. During a 3-hour search in the *Journal of Hospital Infection*, I found the following facts and statements:

- Hand hygiene compliance remains poor[3]
- 54% followed infection control measures only when they perceived an infection threat to themselves[4]
- HCAIs are seen as major safety issues at a global level by the World Health Organization[5]
- It is unlawful for a public body to act incompatibly with a person's rights[6]
- Providers and commissioners of English NHS care are now under a legal obligation to have regard to the NHS Constitution, which establishes a patient's rights[6]
- Compliance with good practices is generally poor[7]
- Staff generally cleaned their hands after clinical examination, presumably because protection of self seems to be the obvious trigger for performing hand hygiene, and not protection of patient.[8]

These are extracts from just one of the many well-respected journals, the very material on which current best practices are based. Could a lawyer argue that current best practices are actually the best *of failed* practices? Around the world, tens of thousands of patients die from HCAIs every year. Might this be why the legal aspects[6] also appear in medical literature? The legal challenge was a major element of the textbook that preceded Elliott's work,[9] So I believe it is well established.

REFLECTION EXERCISE 4

Take a while to determine how often in the previous year those who manage your facilities needed to give due consideration to legal challenges related to poor patient outcomes. Are you able to take action to reduce the incidence of poor outcomes?

So far in this chapter, of the many components of an overall HCAI prevention strategy, only alcohol hand rubs have been discussed. It's fairly easy to see how a lawyer can use the evidence-based research to lead a jury into taking a perspective contrary to that of researchers, health providers and their staff. The latter generated and implemented the data as a means of showing what they believed needed to be improved. If it can be shown they continued to advocate the use of alcohol hand rubs in the face of all this evidence of failure, the jury could be easy to influence. Remember, the excellent points used in the *technical* debate might have little relevance to jurors who learned much of what they know about infections from the media. The press sensationalises the poor *outcome* from hospital infections, so that's where an attacking lawyer could begin. The legal arena is not one where the best *technical* debate wins; it's one where a group of lay jurors could be asked to decide what led to the very poor *outcome* in one specific lethal HCAI case. ICPs have helped compile the published data as they seek to steadily improve outcomes. While the latter is happening, the very same data prove current outcomes are poor and that can only happen if best practices are failing patients who become infected.

Returning to the example of a lethal MSSA infection, the jury could well accept a *technical* statement that alcohol hand rubs kill MSSA. However, this hypothetical court action is only happening because a patient died from MSSA infection. If the alcohol was not to blame, who or what was? A lawyer could make a case that healthcare providers, their management and ICPs head that list.

REFLECTION EXERCISE 5

Give yourself a little space to compare your perspectives with those of your patients and their families. Might you feel their expectations are unrealistic in these times of modern intrusive healthcare? If so, how would you attempt to enhance their appreciation of your realities?

The threat to ICPs is the very evidence-based research they help to compile and publish. That's unfair from the *technical* angle but perfectly justifiable in both the *outcome* and *financial* debates. It's all a matter of perspective.

CHANGE IS SAFER

If researchers, healthcare providers and ICPs continue with current best practices and continue to achieve the same results, they could be targeted with their own data in this manner. For too long, ICPs have concentrated on the *technical* debate and have achieved results that many people, including themselves, consider to be inadequate. That's why they strive to improve patient safety. Rather than abandoning the *technical* debate, they'll benefit from encompassing the *outcome* debate to find a completely different way of addressing the problem. As an example, reframing the patients from being part of the problem to being part of the solution will improve the chances of success. That simple step will reveal ways of positively using all their valuable evidence-based research to protect patients. The first step is that easy. Encompassing the *financial* debate in the same manner makes it even easier, as that adds much needed financial resources.

When ICPs change their perspective and begin to visualise HCAIs as very rare events, they'll find matters evolve quickly. When that happens, this chapter will have achieved the objective of breaking the HCAI cycles. Patients will have helped when they were incorporated into the *who*, but most of the credit will rightly go to ICPs whose new perspective allowed the patients to better defend themselves.

If little changes, most of the blame will continue to be directed at the same profession, and rightly so. Social media is now firmly established. Failure to change in the face of poor outcomes is now more hazardous than change. If you feel embattled, staying where you are while publicly lamenting the poor patient outcomes is the most dangerous option. Since your adversary knows of alternatives that can be argued to be safer for patients and better for staff, you can be asked to explain why you didn't utilise those choices that were clearly available. Citing World Health Organization paperwork and peer-reviewed articles containing evidence-based research will be a weak defence. Remember, if the answers were there, you would be using them and this hypothetical court case would not exist.

Consider another question. If you were forced, in court and under oath, to say whether all the answers needed to end HCAIs were in the medical literature, what would you say? This question is a nasty trap. If you say that the answers are there, you can be asked why you had not utilised them to protect the patient who died. If you say that they are not there, you can be asked to explain why you advised your hospital to use practices that your profession's own evidence has shown were failing many thousands of patients every year.

Now for the good news! Moving on from this trap, and many others like it, requires little effort. The three debates have been presented as separate conflicting entities and the lawyers capitalise on that conflict. When you completely encompass all the debates and overlap them, you'll find enormous resources. Remember that nobody wants the infections, including the lawyers who know how easily they could become patients. They would prefer you to break the HCAI cycles before they encounter them in person.

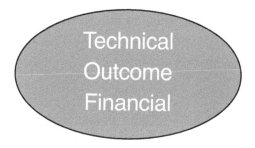

FIGURE 5.2 One single but larger debate in which all the resources are available

Once you genuinely begin to envisage HCAIs being very rare events, you'll have virtually everyone on your side. If you're not genuine and hope to play the public for fools, consider how many people will *not* be on your side. The public now know the choice is between very few infections or thousands of needless HCAI deaths.

SIMPLE ACTIONS

What can be done now to make a real difference?

- Actively challenge paradigms. As an example, is alcohol actually the best choice for hand rubs?
- Test whether your products and practices are fit for purpose. Considering alcohol again, is your primary purpose to follow best practices or to safeguard patients?
- Act on the real problem. Gram-negative bacteria have always been the biggest killers, yet hasn't more effort gone into MRSA because of press coverage?
- Appreciate that reducing infections in the current manner takes time. Consider how long it took to halve the incidence of MRSA infections in Britain. The second is always harder and is likely to take longer. What will you say to a newly bereaved family during that time? Be patient?

- Advance beyond the constraints of best practice and *technical* thinking by also encompassing *outcome* ideas. You will be joining an already active resource of like-minded people known as patients.
- Seek safety in numbers by working with patients and the public. Until then you'll remain the minority, exposed to easy attack.
- Appreciate that healthcare workers' hands are the principal carrier of transient pathogens, so to concentrate on them is to put less emphasis on the source, the patients. Once patients become part of your solution, you're finally addressing the source.
- Consider answers **outside peer-reviewed literature**. You know the answers you need are not all there, or you would be using them. Nor will they be there until people like you ask the appropriate questions. Those questions are frequently asked in the *outcome* debate, accompanied by helpful answers you can easily implement.

The answers you seek are available because the relevant questions have already been asked. Your life would be so much easier if you had those answers among your resources, don't you agree? Virtually everyone wants to be on your side. Wouldn't allowing them to help reduce your anguish and end the lament?

REFERENCES

1. Farmer H. *The Reaper's Rainbow*. Cambridge: NewGenn; 2009.
2. Lampel HP, Patel N, Boyse K, *et al*. Prevalence of hand dermatitis in inpatient nurses at a United States hospital. *Dermatitis*. 2007; **18**(3): 140–2.
3. Smith SJ, Young V, Robertson C, *et al*. Where do hands go? An audit of sequential hand-touch events on a hospital ward. *J Hosp Infect*. 2012; **80**(3): 206–11.
4. Farrugia C, Borg MA. Delivering the infection control message: a communication challenge. *J Hosp Infect*. 2012; **80**(3): 224–8.
5. Cookson B, Mackenzie D, Coutinho AP, *et al*. Consensus standards and performance indicators for prevention and control of healthcare-associated infection in Europe. *J Hosp Infect*. 2011; **79**(3): 260–4.
6. Millar M. Patient rights and healthcare-associated infection. *J Hosp Infect*. 2011; **79**(2): 99–102.
7. Pittet D, Panesar SS, Wilson K, *et al*. Involving the patient to ask about hospital hand hygiene: a National Patient Safety Agency feasibility study. *J Hosp Infect*. 2011; **77**(4): 299–303.
8. Dancer J. Infection control 'undercover': a patient perspective. *J Hosp Infect*. 2012; **80**(3): 189–91.
9. Elliott P, editor. *Infection Control: a psychological approach to changing practice*. Oxford: Radcliffe; 2009.

PART II

Perceptions of infection prevention and control

CHAPTER 6

Stereotyping

. . . .

Paul Elliott

In presenting this chapter my aim is to get you thinking about stereotypes, which will always inevitably be linked to the prejudices and attitudes each of us holds, and of course there consequences to ourselves and others.[1] I will aim to do this both within a general context and specifically with regard to Infection Prevention and Control (IP&C). It is my further intention that this chapter will not be excessively academic in nature but, rather, thought provoking.

LIST 6.1 Everyday stereotypical situations

Consider the following examples.

- You are in a supermarket waiting in line to check your goods out but the person in front of you is moving slowly and not packing their goods as quickly as you would wish or as quickly as you would expect them to do. Do you become frustrated at this? If this has been the case consider what thoughts you may have had about this individual. What perhaps have you muttered about them under your breath or to someone who may be with you in the queue?

- Have you ever seen another individual behave in a certain way that, to you, made no sense or may even have seemed completely bizarre? If this has been the case, what determinations did you make about this person?

- Have you ever been driving a motor vehicle and another individual has done something to distract you or has caused you to feel, shall we say, somewhat upset? What was your reaction?

So, to start with I would like to ask you to think about and make a list of stereotypes you hold. Should you start by questioning whether or not you have any, you are frankly fooling yourself! Everyone has and applies stereotypes in their day-to-day life as a way of helping them to make sense of the world within which they interact (List 6.1).

Whatever your reaction to the examples in List 6.1, they will have been drawn from stereotypes and are likely to have been insulting and/or derogatory (List 6.2).

LIST 6.2 Stereotypical reactions

- Supermarket:
  — *For goodness sake get a move on! Silly old fool!*
  — *People who pack that slowly should be in care!*
- Bizarre behaviour:
  — *What an idiot!*
  — *Are they thick or something!*
- Motor vehicle:
  — Perhaps in this situation you composed a string of short singular words or made reference to certain aspects of the individual's anatomy!
  — Perhaps in this situation you chose to elicit certain hand gestures that may involve a number of fingers!

In considering this, a question I would pose is: how do you define, for example, the terms fool, thick or, for that matter, making reference to the individual's anatomy in a derogatory way? With regard to each of these I would suggest they are connotations related to the notion of an individual's intelligence.[2]

At this point I would like to ask you to write down, without referring to any literature or seeking another's opinion, your definition of intelligence. Having done this please take some time to reflect upon whether you perceive intelligence to be a single characteristic or a range of multiple characteristics and then read on.

In reality intelligence is not something that can or should ever be defined in a singular way,[3] as is the case with that contained within List 6.2. Even intelligence quotient tests, which are taken by some as objective measures of an individual's intelligence, should only at best ever be perceived as a subjective guide, as there remains much debate regarding what such tests actually measure and whether or not they truly measure human intelligence at all.[4]

Arguably intelligence can be perceived as many different things in relation to the

LIST 6.3 Variables that serve to facilitate stereotyping

1. We tend to accept and rationalise[6] in a cognitively economic way[7] what is set before us in a subjective as opposed to an objective way. Where the concepts of subjectivity and objectivity are concerned I would suggest to you that humans are incapable of being objective about anything. Why? Because an individual's perception of the behaviours of others is and will always be drawn from their own past experiences, which may differ from the experiences of the individual they are applying a stereotype to.

2. Each individual's perception or definition of what constitutes intelligent behaviour can be as broad as it may be long. For example, with regard to the speed at which one individual is able to pack their goods in a supermarket queue is not indicative of the speed at which another could or is able do so. Nor is the ability to pack goods in any way a good measure of intelligence. Yet, this is a classic situation where individuals will be likely to apply their concept of intelligence or lack of it to others through the stereotypes they invoke.

3. The beliefs an individual holds about what should or should not constitute normal behaviour is likely to facilitate the application of stereotypes. However, these can be highly subjective, in that where the concept of normality is concerned there is no universal definition. Yet, in observing the behaviour of others one of the ways in which we make sense of such is by drawing upon our beliefs. For example, behaviour taken within a health or social care context can lead health and social care professionals to make decisions based upon what they observe others doing, which in turn tends to lead to the formulation of a belief about a given individual. However, such beliefs are likely to be intuitively based (Figure 6.1) and also drawn from stereotypes that the health or social care professional holds. However, such beliefs are arguably a consequence of our prior learning, which can, for example, be family, culturally, peer group or professionally based. The other point I would make about beliefs and their ability to facilitate the application of stereotypes is that human observation of any kind is highly suspect. A classic example of this is related to what is known as eyewitness testimony.[8] For example, if you and a colleague were to observe the exact same event together at exactly the same moment in time, how likely would it be that you would both relate what you saw in exactly the same way with the same degree of accuracy? The chances of this happening would be questionable.[8] Thus the application of stereotypes through what we observe are generally unreliable in making judgements about others. A very good way of thinking about this is through

an adaptation of the Cognitive Continuum 9 (Figure 6.1), where beliefs and stereotypes would be intuitive (Level 6). Any judgements or decisions that are formulated on intuition alone are neither valid nor reliable, and where infection prevention and control is concerned would be inherently unsafe.

knowledge and/or skills an individual possesses.[5] Further, it could be argued that types of intelligence are infinite with each individual's range of intelligences being multiple and unique to them.[5] Where intelligence and an individual's behaviour are concerned, that individual's behaviour is arguably never random but is always the result of a given stimulus resulting from a physiological, psychological or social experience. In the case of the examples set out within List 6.1, those individuals would have behaved in the way they did for a reason. However, just because others cannot determine that reason or it is not immediately apparent, the application of stereotypes, which may serve to ridicule or be prejudicial of a person's intelligence, are not warranted. As such, instead of stereotyping individuals, what we ought to do is look beyond the obvious and pose the question, why? The problem is of course that human nature is such that with regard to looking beyond the obvious there are three variables that could serve to restrict this (*see* List 6.3).

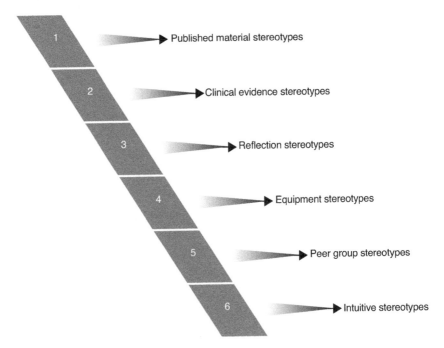

FIGURE 6.1 The Stereotype Continuum[9]

In essence, where stereotypes are concerned one individual's intelligence is arguably another's stupidity, with the stupidity element generally being related to the individual expressing a stereotype.

CLARIFICATION OF LEVELS WITHIN FIGURE 6.1

Level 1

To accept without question what is published as correct and/or will make an effective contribution to the practice of IP&C is to adopt a stereotypical perspective. For example, to assume that a journal where something is published is indicative of an article's quality and its potential for facilitating safe practice is arguably not only a stereotypical perspective but also indicative of intuitive level thinking and decision making. It is the content and applicability to the provision of good, safe, health and social care intervention that matters and not where it has been published, or for that matter who wrote it. From a safe practice perspective, I would argue that if a publication has no application to the real world of IP&C it is of questionable value.

Level 2

To accept without question that because a clinical procedure has always worked in the past it will continue to work and be safe constitutes a stereotypical perspective. With regard to IP&C, the chain of infection has been colloquially accepted as a valid and reliable measure for assessing the risks of cross-infection. Yet, I would argue that such acceptance is inherently flawed, because there appear to be no empirically based findings to support either the development of this chain or to what degree it contributes to any reductions in cross-infection. Further, this chain only tells one-third of the story where the assessing of cross-infection risks are concerned. Thus the continued acceptance of the chain of infection in its current format does in itself constitute a stereotype, because it fails to recognise the psychological and social factors that constitute the other two-thirds of the story and which will also contribute to the potential for cross-infection to occur.[5]

The chain of infection

- Infectious agent
- Reservoirs
- Portals of entry
- Portals of exit

- Susceptible host
- Mode of transmission

Level 3

Reflection is by its nature a subjective process whether it be in action or on action, and as such it is likely to be subject to stereotypical influences. If a practitioner were to rely simply upon their reflective thoughts, judgements and decisions, this would inevitably increase the risk of questionable IP&C practice. NB: Reflection that is in action is where an individual is reflecting as event occurs in real time. Reflection that is on action is where the individual is reflecting after the event has occurred.

Level 4

Equipment is designed and produced by people who are both human and fallible and can therefore have the potential to fail and/or provide unreliable protection where infection prevention and control is concerned. For example, there is published literature to indicate that hand hygiene should be undertaken both before and after the wearing of gloves[10] because as a piece of equipment they may not guarantee 100% protection. However, it is notable that Rock *et al.*[11] appears to suggest that hand hygiene before the application of gloves may not always be necessary in some situations. However, a potential counterargument to this could be that contamination is not unidirectional in its flow but multidirectional, in that it can be passed both ways, between practitioner and other individuals and vice versa. Choosing not to undertake hand hygiene before putting gloves on would seem not to take account of any contamination already on the hands of the practitioner. Although the evidence presented by Rock *et al.*[11] is interesting, my concern would be that such a view could lead to intuitive-level decision making (Figure 6.1) and complacency, which could in turn lead to an increased risk of cross-infection. In essence it should never be assumed that a piece of equipment will give 100% protection where the potential for cross-infection is concerned.

Level 5

Infection prevention and control practitioners transmit large amounts of information, verbally, non-verbally or in writing between one another. Yet, what has to be remembered is that when the transfer of such information takes place, stereotypes are likely to come into play. When passing information on, the individual will transmit the information that they believe is relevant and what others

ought to know. However, what the individual thinks others ought to know is not necessarily what others really **need** to know. For example, cast your mind back to an interaction where you were receiving information from a colleague about a patient and initially it seemed that you had been provided with all relevant information. However, when you encountered the patient it very quickly became evident that you had in fact not been given all relevant information but that there were gaps in what you had been told. Thus the individual giving you the information had stereotyped what they perceived was important and you ought to know about the patient. Based upon the information you had been given, you would have started to determine what you perceived your role to be with the patient until you realised that you had not been given all the information. Subsequently you then had to cognitively reappraise the situation to reduce the potential for harm or cross-infection to occur.

Level 6

Intuition, or gut feeling as it is more often referred to, has the same subjective stereotypical potential as reflection, except to a greater degree where the instigation of safe IP&C practice is concerned. In essence, intuition or gut feeling could be described as, in the absence of objective evidence, making it up as you go along! For example, although the feelings we have may be drawn from past experience (our knowledge base) to apply such in isolation would serve to constitute a stereotypical approach to IP&C practice based on the assumption by an individual that their knowledge base is up to date, correct and safe which, of course, is not always the case.

Summary

Each of Levels 1–6 (Figure 6.1) taken in isolation can only be perceived as serving to facilitate unsafe IP&C practice. What every practitioner should do where IP&C is concerned is to take each of the 6 levels, as the word continuum indicates. Thus, practitioners should be combining and applying several levels at the same time, while moving up and down all levels of the continuum on a continual basis, if their practice is to be potentially safe.

Where individuals have applied stereotypes either intentionally or in the heat of the moment they may, following such, experience feelings of stress, anxiety, anger, embarrassment or fear of retribution and will thus attempt to justify such stereotypes through dissonance-based rationalisations.[5,12] For example, if you were to witness an incident or accident where an individual was clearly in need of your professional intervention but you chose not to make such an intervention and to simply pass by or ignore the situation, you might, if recognised, find yourself subject to investigation from your professional or regulatory body as a result of an act of omission on your part. In reflecting upon this in terms of Freud's model of the human psyche (Figure 6.2), your Id (your basic desires – what you wanted to do or did) would be in conflict with your Superego (your moral conscience – knowing what you should

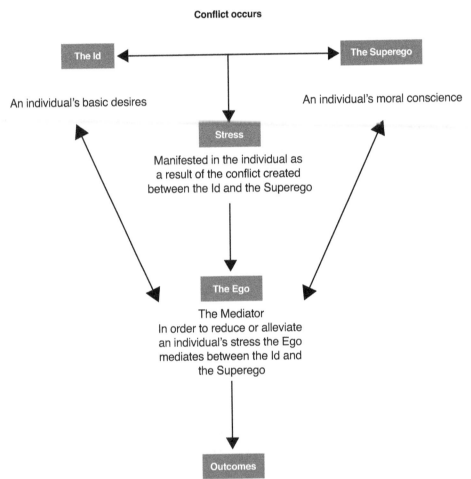

Conflict occurs

The Id

The Superego

An individual's basic desires

An individual's moral conscience

Stress

Manifested in the individual as
a result of the conflict created
between the Id and the Superego

The Ego

The Mediator
In order to reduce or alleviate
an individual's stress the Ego
mediates between the Id and
the Superego

Outcomes

This mediation process can result in a number of potential outcomes:
Rationalised as opposed to rational excuses
Intuitive stereotypes
Unrealistic beliefs
Prejudicial attitudes

FIGURE 6.2 A model of the human psyche (adapted from Atkinson *et al.*, 2011)[13]

have done) and would arguably be manifested as feelings of stress. Therefore, in striving to alleviate any degree of stress you might experience, your Ego (the mediator between your Id and Superego) would seek to resolve such conflict that exists, through the establishment of excuses for failing to act within the confines of your professional code of conduct and moral duty that to you might seem quite acceptable but to others could well be perceived as questionable (List 6.4).

LIST 6.4 Stereotypical excuses for failing to help out

- I didn't stop because I might catch something!
- I couldn't find anywhere to park!
- I expect the paramedics will arrive soon!
- It's not part of my job description!
- I can't be expected to do everything!
- Oh well, I'm sure they're alright!
- I know I should've helped but anyway, I'm sure no one will have noticed or recognised me!
- I know I should've helped but what could I have done? I had nothing with me!
- Who cares! Probably their own fault anyway!
- They're probably just fooling about, it's got to be a hoax!

At this point, consider if you have ever passed by an incident of any sort where you knew full well you ought to have intervened but did not. How did you feel afterward? What excuses did you come up with? How consistent were any excuses you arrived at with your given code of professional conduct or, for that matter, the expectations of society in general?

Inevitably the making of a derogatory statement, gesture or act of omission must be perceived as unprofessional, overtly prejudicial and not consistent with the public perception or the expectations of any professional organisation to which you may be affiliated. Further, such cognitively economic[7] determinations are in essence heuristics (colloquially known as rules of thumb)[14] emanating from, for the most part, very limited information, and as such they will inevitably be underpinned by stereotypical inferences (snap judgements about people, places or objects).

From my own experience of applying heuristics and stereotypical inferences many years ago as a part of my professional role, I encountered an individual whom I perceived as being clearly homeless (a stereotype in itself for which I was wholly guilty). As the department within which I was working was quiet, and having given the individual something to eat and a warm drink, we got chatting, during which a number of stereotypes came to mind: smelly, dirty, possibly infectious and a bit thick (I now look back on these determinations with much shame – they were not only prejudicial but also reflective of what I perceived this individual's intelligence to be). However, as our conversation progressed I became aware that this individual knew a great deal about healthcare and, in particular, medicine. It subsequently transpired that this individual used to be on the British Medical Association's Register of Medical Doctors, which took me completely by surprise and I found myself thinking, why would such a person let themselves come to this? (The asking of such a question was in itself representative of stereotypical thinking). However, what this individual relayed to me was that they had simply reached the point where they could no longer tolerate the stress and excessive working hours of their role. They had therefore made a conscious decision to drop out, as this individual described it. They went on to say that they now had no stress, had made many friends within the homeless community and had a little money each week to help them out. For me this was a defining moment, in that I have never thought about homeless people in the same way since. This experience made me realise that the stereotypes I held at that time were fundamentally prejudicial. However, that is not to say I no longer hold stereotypes. Like everyone else, of course I do! However, since this experience, what I have tried to do is to be less judgemental and to look beyond the obvious. With regards to this particular situation what I did was to apply subjective labels prior to ascertaining the facts of the situation which in reality is what people tend to do as a way of making sense of a situation they do not fully understand or are not fully conversant with.

Within the context of health and social care, the application of labels is something that occurs at an institutional level. For example, let us consider the word 'patient'. It is taken from the Latin *patior*,[15] which means to bear and/or suffer. So when we apply the label patient to those who seek our intervention, what are we actually saying or implying? Are we saying that these people who place their trust and lives in our hands are there to suffer, and having suffered, then have to bear the consequences of our actions or omissions? Such a view taken within the context of IP&C might be perceived as having some relevance. For example, the failure to undertake appropriate standard precautions, which then leads to an individual contracting an infection that they did not have prior to seeking our intervention, clearly means that they will suffer something that they did not have when they entered into our care and which might have been prevented. A point in case being the failure to undertake hand hygiene correctly or at all, when there is a wealth of evidence to support this practice.[16-19] Thus when an individual contracts a healthcare-associated infection through no fault of their own, it may be that the word patient as a stereotype reflects its meaning in the truest sense of its original Latin meaning. Further, the word patient is a clear stereotype that we use to deny people their individuality, and yet we speak much about the importance of maintaining individuality under the guise of person-centred care.[20]

So, in continuing to reflect upon stereotypes and their impact upon IP&C practice and outcomes it is vital to remember that the stereotypes we hold and apply may well serve to increase the risks of cross-infection, reduce adherence to IP&C policy and procedure, such as standard precautions, and have a negative impact upon the way individuals perceive IP&C[5] as an overall measure for not only promoting health and wellbeing but also maintaining the right to life of others.[21]

Arguably, the quality of our IP&C practice is influenced by the attitudes and beliefs we hold or those enforced upon us by others, and the subsequent stereotypes we apply. For example, with regard to the way we practise IP&C, or not, as the case may be, let us consider the notion of truth in relation to what each of us believes constitutes safe and appropriate practice. However, in starting to consider this concept perhaps we should ask the question, what is truth?[22]

At this point what I would ask you to do is write down on a piece of paper something that you believe to be absolutely true. Having done that, ask yourself: How do I know what I have written down is absolutely true? As an example, you might have written down, I am a safe practitioner! But, what evidence can you provide to objectively justify this? (List 6.5 for what you might say.)

LIST 6.5 You might say

- *I always adopt appropriate standard precautions!*
  —But could you recite these if asked? My point being: if you cannot recite them, how can you be sure you are really adopting what constitutes standard precautions? Thus is it really true that you always adopt such?
- *I have never cross-infected anyone!*
  —Are you sure? Just because you believe this does not make it true. It may be that a link between what you did or did not do and an individual or number of individuals who contracted an infection has never been established. You may just have been lucky enough not to have got caught or identified as the culprit!
- *I have always adopted appropriate hand hygiene!*
  —Are you sure? Do you know what appropriate hand hygiene is? If you think

it is hand washing then you are completely wrong! Why? Because washing is only one of the six stages of the hand hygiene process.

— Stage 1 – recognising the need to adopt hand hygiene

— Stage 2 – wet the areas to be washed

— Stage 3 – apply the cleansing solution

— Stage 4 – wash the areas to be cleansed

— Stage 5 – rinse the areas washed thoroughly

— Stage 6 – completely and thoroughly dry the areas rinsed.[5]

- *People thank me!*

  — How do you know they were being truthful? They may just be saying this because they think they will get a better quality of care from you? The truth of what they really believe may be quite different.

- *My colleagues tell me so!*

  — They may say this because they perceive you as being powerful or they may be afraid of you. Or they may tell you this because it is the easiest way out of what might be an embarrassing or confrontational situation.

- *I have never made a mistake!*

  — Who says so? You, so what! You may just be being cognitively economic[7] and suffering from dissonance effects.[5,6] Thus your perception of what constitutes a mistake may be affected as a result of a rationalised, as opposed to rational, perspective.

- *My level of seniority, appointment or experience simply precludes the possibility of my causing cross-infection, because I am an expert!*

  — Really! Such an attitude is more likely to result in cross-infection occurring as a result of an egocentric and egotistical perception of one's own importance. In essence, no one is above causing cross-infection. We all have the potential to do so. Such an attitude might be indicative of an individual having been promoted to the level of their incompetence.

With regard to the examples within List 6.5, these are beliefs that individuals might hold and honestly believe to be true. However, let's consider the following example from List 6.5: 'I have always adopted appropriate hand hygiene!' A good number of years ago I presented a paper at an international IP&C conference. Having introduced myself, I posed the following question to the audience:

In absolute honesty, as professionals, put your hand up if you have always undertaken hand hygiene as well as you knew you should have done.

The reaction was, to say the least, surprising, as not one person in the audience raised their hand. At that point, a clear and audible rumble went across the room. The implication being that in the past these individuals had constituted a clear cross-infection risk through failing to undertake appropriate hand hygiene. Yet, when individuals spoke to me following the presentation they all, without exception, said that until that moment they believed they always had adopted appropriate hand hygiene and were shocked to realise that their belief was not true. With regard to such beliefs and the nature of truth, they are all likely to have been established through and/or influenced by stereotypes these individuals believed made their IP&C behaviour safe and appropriate. So, believing our practice is safe and appropriate does not necessarily make it factually true, and as such it constitutes a misnomer between reality and our subject perception. Where such a misnomer exists it will inevitably enhance the potential for stereotypes being applied and for unsafe IP&C to occur.

Where IP&C is concerned, we as health and social care professionals need to be continuously aware of the stereotypes we apply, the context in which we apply them and be alert to the consequences that their application can have upon ourselves and others. The essential point is that we all have beliefs, attitudes and prejudices that are manifested in the form of stereotypes, and we apply these on a continual basis in order to help us make sense of the world we live in. In many ways these stereotypes are ego-related defence mechanisms that enable us to justify and make sense of the people and objects we encounter and the environments in which we exist as a part of our professional lives and our activities of living.[23] Stereotypes are an integral part of each of us as human beings and they allow us to draw conclusions that to us on an individual basis make perfect sense but which may not necessarily make sense to others. For the most part, the stereotypes we apply are purely intuitive in nature (Figure 6.1) and inherently unreliable, and as such they can serve to facilitate dangerous attitudes and beliefs within a biomedical context[24] leading to physical, psychological and/or social harm being caused to others.

So, in concluding it is my hope that having read through this chapter your understanding and, perhaps more important, your awareness of stereotypes has been enhanced. It is also my hope that in the future you will have a greater awareness of the way you apply them and that you perhaps think twice before you do so.

Having concluded this chapter, I would like to say a few words in memory of a friend and colleague, Professor Melanie Jasper, who is sadly no longer with us. I knew Melanie for many years and had nothing but the highest respect and regard for her. It is my opinion that Melanie was an international leader within the profession of Nursing and that her passing is a great loss to not only the profession of Nursing but healthcare overall. Melanie, you will be missed.

REFERENCES

1. Stapel D, Lindenberg S. Coping with chaos: how disordered contexts promote stereotyping and discrimination. *Science*. 2011; **332**(6026): 251–3.
2. Legg s, Hutter M. *A Collection of Definitions of Intelligence*. 2007. Technical Report. Available at: http://arxiv.org/pdf/0706.3639.pdf (accessed 9 January 2015).
3. Gilman L. The theory of multiple intelligences. Human Intelligence: historical influences, current controversies. *Teaching Resources*. 2001. Available at: www.indiana.edu/~intell/mitheory.shtml (accessed 9 January 2015).
4. Richardson K. What IQ tests test. *Theory Psychol*. 2002; **12**(3): 283–314.
5. Elliott P, editor. *Infection Control: a psychosocial approach to changing practice*. Abingdon: Radcliffe; 2009. pp. 53–7, 235–6.
6. Elliott P. Recognising the psychosocial issues involved in hand hygiene. *J R Soc Promo Health*. 2003; **123**(2): 12–14, 88–94.
7. Roth I, Frisby J. *Perception and Representation: a cognitive approach*. Milton Keynes: Open University; 1992. p. 22.
8. Tversky B, Fisher G. *The Problem with Eyewitness Testimony*. Stanford, CA: Stanford Journal of Legal Studies; 1999. Available at: http://agora.stanford.edu/sjls/Issue%20One/fisher&tversky.htm (accessed 9 January 2015).
9. Hamm RM. Clinical intuition and clinical analysis: expertise and the cognitive continuum. In: Dowie J, Elstein A, editors. *Professional Judgement: a reader in clinical decision making*. Cambridge: Cambridge University Press; 1996. pp. 78–105.
10. *Glove Use for Healthcare Workers*. Heidelberg, Victoria: Hand Hygiene Australia; 2014. Available at: www.hha.org.au/About/GloveUsePolicy.aspx (accessed 9 January 2015).
11. Rock C, Harris A, Reich N, *et al.* Is hand hygiene before putting on nonsterile gloves in the intensive care unit a waste of health care worker time? A randomized controlled trial. *Am J Infect Control*. 2013; **41**(11): 994–6.
12. Festinger L. Cognitive dissonance. *Sci Am*. 1962; **207**(4): 93–102.
13. Atkinson S, Tomley S, Landau C, *et al.*, editors. *The Psychology Book*. London: DK Penguin Group; 2011. pp. 95–7.
14. Shah A, Oppenheimer D. Heuristics made easy: an effort-reduction framework. *Psychol Bull*. 2008; **134**(2): 207–22.
15. Neuberger J. Do we need a new word for patients? *BMJ*. 1999; **318**(7200): 1756–8.
16. Rickard N. Hand hygiene: promoting compliance among nurses and health workers. *Br J Nurs*. 2004; **13**(7): 404–10.

17. Randle J, Clarke J, Storr J. Hand hygiene compliance in healthcare workers. *J Hosp Infect.* 2006; **64**(3): 205–9.

18. Al-Hussami M, Darawad M. Compliance of nursing students with infection prevention precautions: effectiveness of a teaching programme. *Am J Infect Control.* 2013; **41**(4): 332–6.

19. Ataei B, Zahraei S, Pezeshki Z, *et al.* Baseline evaluation of hand hygiene compliance in three major hospitals, Isfahan, Iran. *J Hosp Infect.* 2013; **85**(1): 69–72.

20. Kouble G, Bungay H. *The Challenge of Person-Centred Care: an interprofessional perspective.* Basingstoke: Palgrave Macmillan; 2009. pp. 29–50.

21. Wilkinson R, Caulfield H. *The Human Rights Act: a practical guide for nurses.* London: Whurr; 2001. p. 25.

22. Davidson D. Truth. *Int J Psychoanal.* 2004; **85**(Pt. 5): 1225–30.

23. *Planning Care and Documentation.* London: King's College London; n.d. Available at: http://keats.kcl.ac.uk/pluginfile.php/801606/mod_resource/content/2/page_08.htm (accessed 9 January 2015).

24. Ogden J. *Health Psychology: a textbook.* 5th ed. Maidenhead: McGraw-Hill/Open University Press; 2012. pp. 4–8.

CHAPTER 7

Out-of-hospital infection prevention and control: a paramedic perspective – could we do better?

. . . .

Paul Vigar

It is 3.30 a.m.; Julie is a paramedic treating a patient who has crashed his motorcycle into some metal railings outside of a school and impaled his right leg on one of the railings. It is cold and raining heavily.

The patient is in a great deal of pain and has been bleeding heavily. While firefighters prepare their equipment, Julie prepares to administer intravenous fluids and analgesia to her patient. She is wearing her high-visibility jacket, waterproof trousers, a helmet and a pair of nitrile gloves. She considers the potential for infection in this incident and how she can minimise the risks, given her personal protective equipment and environment. She can't help thinking that this would be much easier in hospital!

INTRODUCTION

Out-of-hospital clinical practice has an important role to play in reducing morbidity and mortality due to healthcare-associated infections, and every practitioner[*] working in this setting has the potential to reduce the risk of infection by operating

---

[*] The term 'practitioner' in this chapter refers to any clinician or healthcare professional and does not specifically refer to a specialist practitioner role such as that of the 'paramedic practitioner'.

consistently within best practice guidelines.[1] A no-tolerance attitude to preventable healthcare-associated infections is now prevalent in the National Health Service.[2]

Outside of hospital, however, more complex care is now being delivered[2] and this presents unique challenges for infection prevention and control; this has led to new, innovative ways of working, contributing to safer practice and reduced hospital stays for patients.

This chapter uses the paramedic role to explore the key issues of infection prevention and control in the out-of-hospital setting at a time when there has been a significant shift in its status, but the principles can be applied to any practitioner working in this environment, including doctors, nurses, physiotherapists, health visitors, occupational therapists, social workers and healthcare support workers.

One of the cornerstones of out-of-hospital infection prevention and control in the emergency setting is the treating of all body fluids as potentially infectious, as the health status of most patients is unknown. It is vital that practitioners working in the out-of-hospital environment have high regard for their own personal hygiene, carefully manage interactions with patients and adequately maintain equipment that may become contaminated with potentially infectious organisms, organic matter or chemicals. Practitioners inevitably have more control over any given situation, leaving their patients at a much greater risk of contracting an infection than themselves, but recent guidance places some responsibility with patients too.[2]

Despite the high risk of exposure to infectious disease, in my experience, knowledge of the aetiology and transmission of infectious disease has been poor and vehicles have not been as clean as patients might expect. Factors such as the appointment of specialist infection control leads, higher education, new equipment, ambulance design and central depots for the cleaning and maintenance of vehicles and equipment are going some way to address a poor record of out-of-hospital infection prevention and control.

REFLECTION EXERCISE 7.1

There is a new pandemic flu virus that has reached the United Kingdom. You are a practitioner who has been asked to assess a 53-year-old woman in her home who has a fever and a cough.

- When do you start thinking about infection prevention and control?
- How might you adapt procedures used in hospital to the out-of-hospital environment?
- How could you protect yourself from potentially becoming infected?

RISK ASSESSMENT

Issues around the prevention and control of infection should be a part of any dynamic risk assessment in the out-of-hospital setting and should begin with information that is received about the call, such as the presenting signs and symptoms of the patient, information from family members or other healthcare professionals and details of the environment. This information could trigger the need for personal protective equipment (PPE) and will contribute to the management of the patient.

The Department of Health highlights three key high-risk areas for the transfer of infection to patients in the pre-hospital setting: (1) direct contact with hands, (2) invasive devices such as cannulas and (3) the emergency environment.[1]

REFLECTION EXERCISE 7.2

You have been called to the scene of a road traffic collision involving two cars and a lorry. There are four patients to manage: three of the patients are still in their cars and one has been ejected from his vehicle and is lying in the road. You have requested further resources but in the meantime you must triage the patients and deliver any lifesaving treatment.

- What kind of PPE should you be wearing?
- How might PPE compromise your ability to adhere to infection prevention and control guidelines?
- From an infection prevention and control perspective, what considerations should be given to assessing four patients in close proximity?

PERSONAL HYGIENE

Healthy skin is an effective barrier to microorganisms, and so breaks in the skin should be covered to minimise the risk of pathogenic organisms entering the body via this route.

High standards of personal hygiene are expected by all healthcare professionals, but given that hands are the most common way in which microorganisms might be transported and subsequently cause infection, good hand hygiene* is the single most important method for minimising the risk of infections.[1] Studies have shown that a nurse's hands can be contaminated during even clean procedures such as lifting patients and performing patient observations.[3] Paramedics are constantly in contact with their patient, the surrounding environment, the ambulance and

---

* Hand hygiene comprises both hand washing with water and a cleansing solution and the use of hand rubs.

equipment, yet access to hand hygiene facilities in the out-of-hospital environment is challenging. However, the move over recent years from hand washing to hand rub with alcohol-based preparations under certain conditions has revolutionised hand hygiene practices.[4]

The World Health Organization describes the five moments of hand hygiene[3] and the National Patient Safety Agency has provided a number of resources focusing on non-ward-based care (*see* Figures 7.1, 7.2 and 7.3).[5]

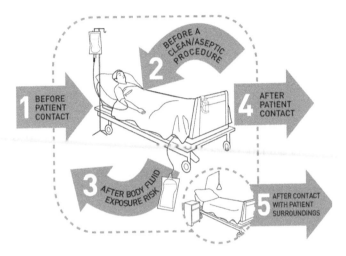

FIGURE 7.1 The five moments of hand hygiene (National Patient Safety Agency[5]) Reproduced with the permission of the WHO from *Five Moments of Hand Hygiene*.

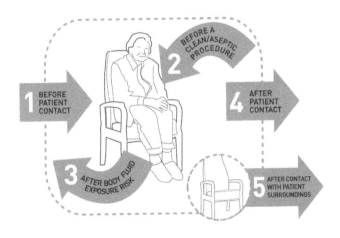

FIGURE 7.2 The five moments of hand hygiene (National Patient Safety Agency[5]) Reproduced with the permission of the WHO from *Five Moments of Hand Hygiene*.

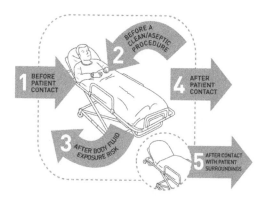

FIGURE 7.3 The five moments of hand hygiene (National Patient Safety Agency[5])
Reproduced with the permission of the WHO from *Five Moments of Hand Hygiene*.

REFLECTION EXERCISE 7.3

Have a think about the five moments of hand hygiene described by the World Health Organization[3] and illustrated in Figures 7.1, 7.2 and 7.3. Consider some of the practical challenges of working outside of the hospital environment.

BOX 7.1 Challenges of hand hygiene in the out-of-hospital setting

- The patient's medical history or history of presenting complaint may be unknown.
- You may have just got out of a vehicle: you may have been using communication equipment; you may have been driving, putting you in contact with vehicle controls; and you would have touched the outside of the vehicle.
- You may have to carry equipment to the patient.
- There may be a need for an immediate assessment or action in an emergency.
- The patient may require time-critical, invasive interventions.
- Access to hand-washing facilities may be limited, e.g. at the scene of a car accident or an assault in the high street, or in a dirty environment.
- Hand-washing facilities may be inadequate, e.g. at a patient's home.

Hands that are visibly soiled must be washed with soap and water,[3] which may not be available in the out-of-hospital setting. Even if hand-washing facilities are available, the quality will vary given that the majority of locations will be patients' homes.

While it would be possible to install running water and sinks in an ambulance, the availability of sinks is not considered a priority by the World Health Organization,[3] especially when there are limited resources and many practitioners will not be working in an ambulance. In the absence of soap and water, detergent wipes can be used followed by alcohol gel once the hands are dry.[1] However, there is little evidence on the clinical and cost-effectiveness of such alternatives.[2] Detergent wipes could be stored in response bags to further increase compliance at the patient's side when hands are soiled, and alcohol hand rubs are now widely available.

It is my experience that compliance with hand hygiene techniques outside of hospital is poor but there is little credible research in this specific setting. It is likely that reasons for poor compliance out of hospital will be the same as in hospital and include poor access to hand hygiene supplies, skin irritation caused by the cleaning agents, interference with the clinician–patient relationship, carelessness, poor knowledge of the guidelines and a lack of time.[3,6]

While it is current practice to only wear gloves when there is a risk of coming into contact with blood and other body fluids, it is my experience that some practitioners working out of hospital wear gloves while performing other tasks such as opening doors and driving. Gloves do not offer complete protection and are no substitute for good hand hygiene, and the prolonged use of gloves can itself result in the transmission of infection.[3]

The World Health Organization explains that artificial acrylic fingernails are associated with poor infection prevention despite the use of soap or alcohol gel.[3] Such nails are often banned under uniform policies but the wearing of plain wedding rings is permitted, despite being associated with an increased frequency of hand contamination.[3]

PERSONAL PROTECTIVE EQUIPMENT

Uniforms are not considered to be protective equipment[7] and there is no conclusive evidence that uniforms play a direct role in spreading infection, but they should minimise risk to patients and be clean.[8] Whether uniform is worn or not, out-of-hospital practitioners should have access to equipment that they can utilise in the event of a potential exposure. The choice of equipment should be based on a risk assessment[7] to include the risk of transmitting microorganisms to the patient[2] or other healthcare workers.[1]

The Department of Health introduced a 'bare below the elbows' policy, which aims to prevent the spread of infection from contaminated sleeves and to facilitate better hand hygiene procedures,[1] but there is a tension between staff comfort in cold, wet environments, health and safety when wearing high-visibility clothing and infection prevention and control. The National Institute for Health and Care Excellence acknowledge that practitioners working outside may have to wear PPE in line with health and safety legislation but that there should be provision for adequate hand decontamination.[2]

PPE could include disposable sterile or non-sterile gloves, plastic aprons, sleeve protectors (when wearing jackets), shoe protectors, paper suits, face masks and safety eyewear. Some emergency workers are now even equipped with respirators for use with patients suspected to be suffering with severe acute respiratory syndrome or in the case of a pandemic flu outbreak.[1,9] Table 7.1 illustrates when PPE should be worn in the out-of-hospital environment.

TABLE 7.1 Personal protective equipment in the out-of-hospital setting*

Personal protective equipment	Reasons to be worn
Gloves	Risk of contact with blood or body fluids
	When sharp or contaminated items are being handled
	Contact with non-intact skin or mucous membranes
	Risk of contamination from blood or body fluids
	Potential contamination from cleaning procedures
	When transporting known infectious patients
Sleeve protector	Protects uniform from wrist to elbow from body fluids and skin cells
Shoe protectors	As for items already listed, if additional protection is required
Paper suit	As for items already listed, if additional protection is required
Face mask	Risk of contact with blood or body fluids from slashes or respiratory droplets
	Risk of inhaling infected respiratory particles
Eye protection	Risk of contact with blood or body fluids from splashes or respiratory droplets
Respirator	Protection against certain respiratory disease (e.g. severe acute respiratory syndrome, pandemic flu)

* Based on information from the Department of Health[1] and Pellowe *et al.*[9]

REFLECTION EXERCISE 7.4

You are a practitioner working on your own in a car and you have been called to a 22-year-old male and a 19-year-old female who have fallen from an off-road motorcycle on a farm. The male patient has fractured his right femur, has a large open wound to his upper right arm with substantial tissue loss, is in a great deal of pain and is unable to move, while the female patient is complaining of a shoulder injury.

- What procedures might you need to carry out that increase the risk of infection for these patients?
- What challenges are there for infection prevention and control in this scenario?
- How can you best minimise the risk of infection when managing these patients?

ASEPTIC TECHNIQUE

Asepsis is defined as the absence of pathogenic organisms, and aseptic technique is a method used to prevent the contamination of the body through clinical procedures.[1] Aseptic technique plays a vital role in preventing the transmission of infection but an adequate sterile field can rarely be achieved outside of hospital, and so a non-touch technique is adopted to include good hand hygiene, the wearing of sterile or non-sterile gloves where appropriate and not touching key parts of items that will be in direct contact with the patient.

Gloves can tear easily, particularly at the scene of road traffic collisions where there might be metal and glass hazards and the majority of products offer little protection against sharps injuries. Where there is more than one casualty, gloves should be changed between patients and before moving onto a new task,[1] but this can be challenging, especially when combined with the use of alcohol hand gel in an emergency situation where time-critical procedures may need to be performed or where you need to assess more than one patient rapidly.

Intravenous cannulation has long been carried out in the out-of-hospital setting by paramedics and other healthcare professionals alike, but it poses a clear infection risk; by definition there is an inherent risk of infection, as the needle provides a direct route for microbes into the patient's bloodstream.[10] The intravenous cannula may be contaminated by the patient's skin flora at the insertion site or by the introduction of other organisms via the cannula hub or injection port.[10] Where intravenous cannulas cannot be inserted aseptically, they are classified as 'emergency inserted', resulting in a replacement cannula being used at the receiving hospital.[1]

Other equipment such as skin preparation applicators containing chlorhexidine gluconate and isopropyl alcohol, sterile cannulation packs and disposable tourniquets are contributing to more effective infection prevention and control when performing intravenous cannulation. Endotracheal intubation is being supported by disposable laryngoscope handles and blades, which are in stark contrast to the reusable equipment in bags available to paramedics in the past and often cleaned in sinks at the hospital after use. Careful attention must be paid to ensuring kit bags are not overstocked, which can cause damage to the packaging of single-use items prior to use.

REFLECTION EXERCISE 7.5

You are working alone in a car and have been asked to attend an elderly lady who has had a fall and has sustained a deep laceration to her left forearm. You decide that the best way to close this wound is using sutures. Your patient lives alone and appears a little unkempt, her flat is dirty and untidy, and she has five cats living with her who use a litter tray.

What can you do to minimise the risk of infection in your management of this patient?

EQUIPMENT AND VEHICLES

Increasingly, equipment bags are made of fabrics with an antibacterial treatment that are easy to wipe clean and patient assessment devices feature disposable parts where there is contact with the patient.

The use of needles in the out-of-hospital setting can be risky, given the unpredictable nature of the environment, the potential for poor light, and so on. Given that the majority of exposures are due to inappropriately discarded needles among allied healthcare professionals,[11] needles that are automatically sheathed or retracted are now in use around the United Kingdom. Sharps bins are generally available in response bags, ambulances and response cars to enable easy access in all manner of scenarios, with sizes varying depending on their location and intended use.

Blood and body fluids, which are considered hazardous, can now be cleaned up with wipes or kits that are now readily available in most UK ambulance services, and when used with the appropriate PPE these contribute to timely management of body fluid spills with a view to reducing the risk of infection to clinical staff, patients and bystanders in public areas, although there is a dearth of research in this area. Ambulances and response cars are equipped with clinical waste bins for the disposal of waste associated with clinical presentations and procedures but there is not always access to non-clinical waste bins.

The cleanliness of premises and vehicles is an important component of the provision of clean, safe care, and the National Health Service Constitution clearly states that services will be provided in a clean and safe environment fit for purpose based on national best practice.[12] While there have been significant improvements in the cleanliness of ambulances over recent years we must not become complacent. Frequent cleaning of vehicles and a weekly deep clean of an ambulance by practitioners used to be commonplace, but the increasing year-on-year demand on ambulance services[13] has compromised this process. In my experience, interior ambulance surfaces have been poorly maintained, with dirt and dust visible to the naked eye in the past, stretchers are rarely wiped, and patient monitoring equipment is not always regularly cleaned between patients to this day.

The availability of cleaning materials, especially surface wipes, together with education has increased compliance with these tasks, but regular cleaning needs to be balanced with the demand and pressure to attend increasing numbers of emergency calls. There are new innovative systems embedding themselves in the United Kingdom now, such as Make Ready, where vehicles are regularly deep cleaned and swabbed for the presence of microorganisms by specialist teams as part of a regular maintenance, cleaning and equipment stocking schedule.[14] In addition, ambulance design is evolving with consideration given to facilitating effective hygiene and infection control including rounded corners, covered joints, separation of clinical and non-clinical waste, sealed drawers, easy-clean seats, removable seatbelts and readily demountable equipment for cleaning.[15]

Most linen has the potential to harbour microorganisms and will be deposited at hospitals for washing, having been segregated into general and contaminated linen bags. Where patients are not being transported to hospital, having been assessed and treated on an ambulance, linen is left on the ambulance until it can be safely disposed of, which can be unsightly and may pose an infection risk to other patients treated in the vehicle prior to safe disposal of the linen. This could easily be resolved with a suitable storage area.

MOVING FORWARD

Everyone providing care in the community should be educated about the standard principles of infection prevention and control and there should be sufficient supplies of equipment available.[2]

Traditionally, infection control training for ambulance staff was minimal, but this limited training has given way to higher education with university paramedic science courses obliged to equip students with the skills to establish and maintain a safe practice environment that minimises the risk to service users and practitioners,[16] and to be aware of local infection control procedures.[17]

Human health-related behaviour is determined by our biology, environment, religion and culture as well as our education,[3] and so all of these factors need to be understood and considered when taking action on improving infection prevention and control behaviours and may be a useful focus for research.

While a zero tolerance approach may be difficult to achieve in the out-of-hospital setting in real terms, to move forward we need effective infection prevention and control measures, a strong commitment from clinical leaders and managers, healthcare-associated infection to become an indicator of the quality and safety of patient care and the provision of quality information to the public as well as clinical staff.[6]

There also needs to be a robust system of monitoring and audit to monitor compliance and drive improvements, which could include financial remuneration through the Commissioning for Quality and Innovation payment framework, which rewards National Health Service organisations for meeting locally agreed quality improvement and innovation goals. However, a recent review identified disappointing results in terms of the impact of this framework on existing goals.[18]

SUMMARY

Reducing the number of healthcare-associated infections is crucial and out-of-hospital practitioners have an important role to play in achieving this goal. Despite the challenges of the working environment and a poor record of managing infection prevention and control outside of hospital, clinical practice is changing.

It is clear that a number of factors contribute to effective infection prevention and control in the out-of-hospital setting discussed in this chapter and illustrated in Figure 7.4; there is a paucity of research relating to many of the key topics raised, but it is apparent that a multifactorial approach is needed to improve current practice and clinical outcomes.

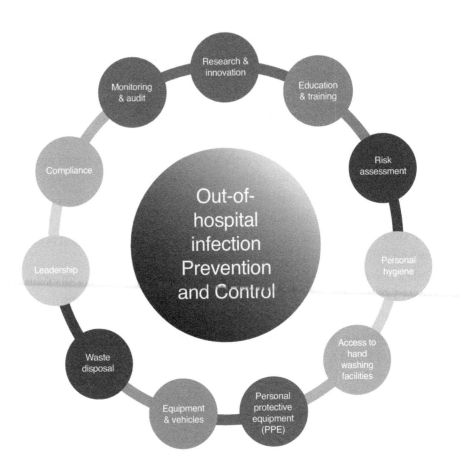

FIGURE 7.4 Key issues for out-of-hospital infection prevention and control

Better education and training, more stringent policies and procedures, effective leadership, new systems of working and access to more appropriate equipment at the right moments of patient care are all contributing to improved infection prevention and control, but there is still some way to go and any action needs to be sustained if changes to clinical practice and behaviour are to be achieved.

Most important, there needs to be more research into issues of infection prevention and control in the out-of-hospital setting, and longer-serving members of staff need to be able to access the same literature as new paramedics in higher education and be motivated to do so. The National Institute for Health and Care Excellence highlights research recommendations that include barriers to compliance, the clinical and cost-effectiveness of using wipes and gels when clean running water is unavailable, and the effectiveness of different substances used for skin decontamination prior to gaining vascular access.[2]

There needs to be much more emphasis on infection control when teaching and assessing clinical skills; further consideration given to how current methods of infection prevention and control can be modified, given that the role of the ambulance service is changing to include the management of patients in their own home; and sharing of good practice.

Finally, systems of monitoring and audit need to be implemented to monitor compliance and identify deficiencies that can be acted on in this battle against healthcare-associated infections.

REFERENCES

1. HCAI and Cleanliness Division, Department of Health. *Ambulance Guidelines: reducing infection through effective practice in the pre-hospital environment.* London: Department of Health; 2008. Available at: http://webarchive.nationalarchives.gov.uk/20130107105354/http://www.dh.gov.uk/prod_consum_dh/groups/dh_digitalassets/@dh/@en/documents/digitalasset/dh_087428.pdf (accessed 2 March 2015).
2. National Institute for Health and Care Excellence. *Infection: prevention and control of healthcare-associated infection in primary and community care: NICE guideline 139.* London: NIHCE; 2012. www.nice.org.uk/guidance/cg139
3. World Health Organization (WHO). *World Health Organization Guidelines on Hand Hygiene in Health Care.* Geneva: WHO; 2009. Available at: http://whqlibdoc.who.int/publications/2009/9789241597906_eng.pdf (accessed 19 June 2012)
4. Boyce J, Pittet D. Guideline for hand hygiene in health-care settings: recommendations of the Healthcare Infection Control Practices Advisory Committee and the HICPAC/SHEA/APIC/IDSA Hand Hygiene Task Force. *Morbidity and Mortality Weekly Report.* 2002; **51**: 1–50. Available at: www.cdc.gov/mmwr/pdf/rr/rr5116.pdf (accessed 30 July 2012)
5. National Patient Safety Agency. *Your Five Moments Explained: hospital non-ward based care.* 2011. Available at: www.npsa.nhs.uk/cleanyourhands/resource-area/nhs-resources/education/training-five-moments/ (accessed: 30 July 2012)
6. Chief Medical Officer. *Winning Ways: working together to reduce healthcare associated infection in England.* London: Department of Health; 2003. Available at: http://webarchive.nationalarchives.gov.uk/20130107105354/http://www.dh.gov.uk/prod_consum_dh/groups/dh_digitalassets/@dh/@en/documents/digitalasset/dh_4064689.pdf (accessed: 2 March 2015)
7. Health and Safety Executive. *Control of Substances Hazardous to Health.* 6th ed. Merseyside: HSE Books; 2013.
8. Department of Health. *Uniforms and Workwear: guidance on uniform and workwear policies for NHS employers.* London: Department of Health; 2010. Available at: http://webarchive.nationalarchives.gov.uk/20130107105354/http://www.dh.gov.uk/prod_consum_dh/groups/dh_digitalassets/@dh/@en/@ps/documents/digitalasset/dh_114754.pdf (accessed 2 March 2015)
9. Pellowe C, Loveday H, Pratt R, *et al.* Standard principles: personal protective equipment and the safe use and disposal of sharps. *Nursing Times.* 2007 Nov 20. Available at: www.nursingtimes.net/nursing-practice/specialisms/management/standard-principles-personal-

protective-equipment-and-the-safe-use-and-disposal-of-sharps/291502.article (accessed 2 March 2015).

10. Department of Health. *High Impact Intervention no. 2. Peripheral intravenous cannula care bundle: saving lives, reducing infection, delivering clean and safe care.* London: Department of Health; 2007. Available at: http://webarchive.nationalarchives.gov.uk/20120118164404/hcai.dh.gov.uk/files/2011/03/2011-03-14-HII-Peripheral-intravenous-cannula-bundle-FIN%E2%80%A6.pdf (accessed 5 January 2014).

11. Health Protection Agency. *Eye of the Needle: surveillance of significant occupational exposure to bloodborne viruses in healthcare workers.* London: HPA; 2008. Available at: http://webarchive.nationalarchives.gov.uk/20140714084352/http://www.hpa.org.uk/webc/HPAwebFile/HPAweb_C/1227688128096 (accessed 2 March 2015).

12. National Health Service. *NHS Constitution.* London: NHS; 2012. Available at: www.nhs.uk/choiceintheNHS/Rightsandpledges/NHSConstitution/Documents/nhs-constitution-interactive-version-march-2012.pdf (accessed 30 July 2012).

13. Association of Ambulance Chief Executives. *Taking Healthcare to the Patient 2: a review of 6 years' progress and recommendations for the future.* Association of Ambulance Chief Executives; 2011.

14. South East Coast Ambulance Service NHS Foundation Trust. *Make Ready.* South East Coast Ambulance Service NHS Foundation Trust; 2013. Available at: www.secamb.nhs.uk/about_us/our_developments/make_ready.aspx (accessed 20 December 2013).

15. The Helen Hamlyn Trust; National Patient Safety Agency. *Design for Patient Safety: future ambulances.* London: The Helen Hamlyn Trust; National Patient Safety Agency; 2007. Available at: www.nrls.npsa.nhs.uk/resources/type/guidance/?entryid45=59816&p=3 (accessed 17 October 2013).

16. Health Professions Council. *Standards of Proficiency: paramedics.* London: Health Professions Council; 2007. Available at: www.hpc-uk.org/assets/documents/1000051CStandards_of_Proficiency_Paramedics.pdf (accessed 30 July 2012).

17. Quality Assurance Agency for Higher Education. *Paramedic Science. Benchmark statement: health care programmes.* Gloucester: Quality Assurance Agency for Higher Education; 2004. Available at: www.qaa.ac.uk/en/Publications/Documents/Subject-benchmark-statement-Health-care-programmes---Paramedic-Science.pdf (accessed 24 July 2012).

18. MacDonald R, Zaidi S, Todd S, *et al. Evaluation of the Commissioning for Quality and Innovation Framework: final report.* 2013. Available at: http://hrep.lshtm.ac.uk/publications/CQUIN_Evaluation_Final_Feb2013-1.pdf (accessed 2 March 2015).

CHAPTER 8

Antibiotics: help or hindrance?

....

Sarah Pye and Clare Hancock

INTRODUCTION

Regardless of the numerous guidelines, extensive research, worldwide media campaigns and public awareness–raising initiatives, antibiotic resistance remains a threat to global public health.[1] This chapter will consider the extent to which bacteria are evading the antibiotic. How bacteria become resistant will be discussed, along with the strategies that are being implemented to combat the rising number of antibiotic-resistant infections.

REFLECTION EXERCISE

Consider why antibiotic resistance occurs. Reflect upon the consequences of antibiotic resistance in healthcare and consider what actions can be taken to reduce the problem. Compare your thoughts with what follows throughout the chapter.

THE EXTENT OF THE PROBLEM

In 2011, over 40 million prescriptions for antibacterial drugs were dispensed in the United Kingdom (UK).[2] Alarming stories about antibiotics are a regular feature of the mass media and recent newspaper headlines have highlighted the antimicrobial resistance (AMR) crisis in healthcare.[3,4] It has been estimated by the European Commission[5] that in the European Union:

- approximately 25 000 patients per year die from drug-resistant bacterial infections
- approximately 4 million patients per year acquire a healthcare-associated infection
- the costs associated with AMR exceed 1.5 billion Euros.

There have been repeated public health campaigns to increase awareness of the risks associated with inappropriate antibiotic prescribing. For example, the annual European Antibiotic Awareness Day coordinated by the European Centre for Disease Prevention and Control aims to raise awareness about the threat to public health of antibiotic resistance, and prudent antibiotic use.

Despite these efforts, recent research by the Health Protection Agency[6] has shown that over half of those visiting their doctor for a respiratory tract infection expected a prescription for an antibiotic. A quarter of people surveyed thought that antibiotics were effective treatment for most coughs and colds.

With rising rates of AMR, the rational and prudent prescribing of antibiotics presents a major challenge for healthcare providers. Consequently, the World Health Organization (WHO) has called this 'a developing global crisis in health care' requiring urgent action to address the problem.[7]

HOW AND WHY DOES ANTIMICROBIAL RESISTANCE DEVELOP?

AMR is not a new phenomenon[8] – resistance was observed within years of antibiotics being available for widespread use. For example, in 1963 ampicillin was introduced as the first broad-spectrum penicillin. At launch it was active against *Escherichia coli* but by 1965 ampicillin-resistant *E. coli* had been discovered.[9]

AMR develops due to the occurrence of genetic mutations, which allow bacteria to resist the action of an antimicrobial agent.[10] Exposure to antibiotics creates an evolutionary pressure that selects for bacteria with resistant traits: an example of Charles Darwin's 'survival of the fittest' evolutionary theory. Inappropriate prescribing and poor adherence to treatment by patients both contribute to the development of AMR.[11]

The use of certain antibacterial treatments can predispose patients to future antimicrobial-resistant infections. For example, *Clostridium difficile* infection often occurs after a patient has received antibiotic treatment.[12] The risk of developing *C. difficile* infection is greatest with ampicillin, amoxicillin, co-amoxiclav, second- and third-generation cephalosporins, clindamycin, and quinolones, but most antibiotics have been associated with this side effect.[12] Patients who have recently received antibiotic treatment, particularly quinolone or macrolide antibiotics, are thought to be at greater risk of developing a meticillin-resistant *Staphylococcus aureus* (MRSA) infection compared to those who have received no antibiotic treatment.[13]

TREATMENT OF ANTIMICROBIAL-RESISTANT INFECTIONS

The management of antimicrobial-resistant infections is a continually changing landscape, with new challenges appearing on a regular basis.[14] The management of MRSA and *C. difficile* infections are well described, but healthcare professionals need to be aware of changing resistance patterns. The emergence of new multi-resistant infections, such extended-spectrum beta-lactamases (ESBLs) and carbapenemase-producing Enterobacteriaceae, to antibiotics is cause for considerable concern, as difficult-to-treat infections have the potential to put significant strain on the healthcare system.

Infections caused by bacteria-producing ESBLs are one example of a difficult-to-treat infection that is on the increase. ESBLs are enzymes that enable the bacteria to resist the action of commonly prescribed antibiotics, such as cephalosporins and penicillins. ESBL infections were discovered in the 1980s and, until relatively recently, were rarely encountered. Risk factors for developing an ESBL infection include serious underlying disease, prolonged hospital stay, presence of invasive medical devices and previous antibiotic usage.[15] Treatment options are limited but include nitrofurantoin, fosfomycin and carbapenems.

Carbapenem antibiotics, such as imipenem and meropenem, have a broad spectrum of activity and are used for the treatment of severe hospital-associated infections and polymicrobial infections.[16] As such they are often used as last-line treatments for resistant infections. Worryingly, carbapenem resistance has begun to develop, resulting in bacteria that are resistant to all but a handful of antibiotics. A growing number of bacteria from the Enterobacteriaceae species, such as *E. coli* and Klebsiella, have been noted to produce carbapenemase enzymes.[17] These enzymes destroy carbapenem antibiotics, and therefore bacteria producing them can cause multidrug-resistant infections.[18] Resulting infections present a therapeutic challenge, as there are limited treatment options, such as colistin and tigecycline.[19] This is has been a growing problem in recent years. The United States, India and parts of Europe are all reported to have high prevalence of healthcare-associated carbapenemase-producing Enterobacteriaceae.[20]

FUTURE DEVELOPMENTS AND NEW ANTIMICROBIAL TREATMENTS

As bacteria have developed resistance to treatment with traditional antibiotics, hope has turned to the development of new drugs to overcome the problem.[21] The complex process of taking new chemical entities from the laboratory bench to the patient, and the significant associated development costs, mean that the supply of new treatments by the pharmaceutical industry has not met the demand in recent years.[7]

Both WHO[22] and the European Commission[23] have called for innovation in antibiotic drug development to help tackle this crisis. WHO[24] has recommended that government incentives should be used to encourage the pharmaceutical industry to invest in research and development for new antimicrobials. It has also suggested that fast-track systems could be developed for medicines regulators to bring new agents to the market.[25]

New antibacterial drugs have reached the market in recent years, but speed of drug development has not matched the demand for new treatments.[26] Some new treatments have failed to live up to expectations. For example, tigecycline was released in 2006 as a treatment for complicated skin and soft tissue, and intra-abdominal infections. In 2011, the Medicines and Healthcare Products Regulatory Agency issued a warning that tigecycline should only be used when other antibiotics are unsuitable, because of increased mortality rates observed in clinical trials.[27] As such, the treatment has a limited value and is not routinely used. The usefulness of newly launched antimicrobial drugs, such as ceftaroline and fidaxomicin, remain to be seen.

The development of AMR is inevitable and we can only act to slow its progress, not eradicate it completely.[28] Due to the rapid replication of bacteria and the associated genetic mutations that lead to AMR, scientific research will always struggle to keep pace. Drug development is unlikely to provide timely solutions, in sufficient volume, to tackle the growing problem of antimicrobial-resistant infections.[29] Therefore, it is essential that existing antimicrobials are used prudently, following local guidance and sensitivity results where these are available, to slow progress of AMR. The many factors that influence the prescribing of antibiotics and can lead to antibiotic misuse shall now be considered.

WHAT DO WE MEAN BY ANTIBIOTIC MISUSE?

> **REFLECTION EXERCISE**
>
> Reflect on what is meant by antibiotic misuse. Compare your thoughts with the discussion outlined in this section.

If prudent prescribing is required, are antibiotics currently prescribed irresponsibly or misused? The link between antibiotic use and resistance is noted, and misuse of antibiotics is indeed considered to be a causative factor in the rise of AMR.[30] If bacteria continue to evade the antibiotic this is a problem that could in fact get worse. WHO recognises this as a global threat and calls for 'stronger action worldwide to avert a situation that entails an ever increasing health and economic burden'.[31] Interventions have been aimed at reducing the risks associated with AMR, including targeted education for the public, health workers and prescriber, and awareness-raising campaigns. These activities span almost 2 decades of intervention, but they have done little, it seems, to reverse the tide. As the most commonly prescribed drug, the way in which antibiotics are used is vital in the fight against antibiotic resistant bacteria. A recent report, *Antibiotic Resistance Threats in the United States, 2013*, from the Centers for Disease Control and Prevention (CDC),[32] states that 'up to 50% of all the antibiotics prescribed for people are not needed or are not optimally effective as prescribed'. From the vast array of published literature, antibiotic misuse could be described as:

- unnecessary prescribing of antibiotics, overuse (e.g. for viral infections)
- use of broad-spectrum antibiotics, or narrow-spectrum antibiotics used incorrectly
- misuse and inappropriate dosing, route of administration and/or treatment duration
- prescribing in the absence of microbiological culture results.

There is evidence to support the view that there is a clear link between antibiotic resistance and the use of antibiotics by patients and prescribers. This evidence is global and spans over a decade.[33–36] It is important that the role of prescribers and the public in tackling this problem is considered. The reported issue of misuse of antibiotics perhaps assumes there is a general belief that there is a problem.[37] However, this may not be the case. There is evidence[38,39] to suggest that not all clinicians or patients see antibiotic resistance as a reason for antibiotics not to be prescribed; some clinicians even view the risk as 'theoretical or minimal' and some state 'the issue has been exaggerated'. It seems interventions are required in the education of both prescribers and the general public. Perhaps a starting point would be to consider why prescriptions are issued in the first place. It could be argued that a prescription is issued to achieve a therapeutic objective, either to:

- relieve a symptom
- reach curative outcome
- or prevent a condition occurring.

In the case of a prescription for an antibiotic, it is apparent that the prescriber should be aiming to reach a curative outcome. This would assume an accurate diagnosis is made, the bacterium causing the infection is known and there is evidence to suggest an antibiotic will cure the infection.

However, there is evidence to suggest that prescribers are not influenced by clinical factors alone when prescribing.[40-45] While an abundance of evidence exists, a systematic review by Lopez-Vazquez[46] warns that some evidence has limited significance due to limitations in methodology, although this review did recognise complacency (patient expectation) and fear (complications) as related to inappropriate prescribing.

WHAT INFLUENCES ANTIBIOTIC PRESCRIBING?

REFLECTION EXERCISE

Reflect upon what you feel may influence antibiotic prescribing and then compare your thoughts with the influences identified in this section.

There is an abundance of evidence to suggest that non-clinical factors are also considered when making the decision to prescribe medication, including antibiotics.[47-54] These factors have been categorised into those relating to the patient and those relating to the prescriber.

Prescriber-related factors include:

- personal characteristics
- knowledge
- features of clinical practice
- prescribing preferences

- local management policies
- patient expectation
- fear of uncertainty about diagnosis, complications, experience
- evidence and policy
- drug companies
- patient demand or satisfaction.

Patient-related factors include:
- socio-economic status
- quality of life
- expectations and wishes
- lack of knowledge
- beliefs of health and illness
- previous treatment with antibiotics.

Macro and micro decisions relating to prescribing practice have been observed in a small study examining variations in prescribing practice among general practitioners (GPs).[55]

Where non-clinical influences on prescribing have an effect on the number of prescriptions for antibiotics, it seems that measures to reduce antibiotic prescribing will need to respond to these factors in addressing the issues highlighted by the World Health Organization[56] and the International Forum on Antibiotic Resistance colloquium.[57] These factors, it would seem, require intervention at several levels. For example, public education is required to raise awareness of the role of antibiotics in disease; prescribers need to be judicious in their decisions to prescribe an antibiotic. These strategies aim to reduce the risks associated with misuse or overuse of antibiotics.

The factors listed earlier could be considered in the context of the following:
- the prescriber–patient relationship
- uncertainty of diagnosis and progression of illness
- lack of knowledge and understanding of the role of antibiotics.

THE PRESCRIBER–PATIENT RELATIONSHIP

There is some evidence to suggest that patients are more likely to be given an antibiotic if they ask for one, or when they exert pressure on the prescriber to prescribe.[58-60]

REFLECTION EXERCISE

Reflect upon why patients may exert pressure on the prescriber to prescribe and compare your thoughts with the suggested list outlined in this section.

- To prove they are ill
- To feel something is being done
- Because they have faith in medicines
- Rather not alter their lifestyle
- Because it has worked before
- To avoid cost of purchasing medicine
- Addiction
- As an alternative to other treatment
- 'Just in case'
- Direct-to-consumer advertising (United States and New Zealand)[61]

Prescriber–patient relationship factors may be linked to the personal characteristics of prescribers or fear of retribution if an antibiotic is not prescribed and the patient becomes more unwell. A study considering the use of broad-spectrum antibiotics found that GPs were likely to prescribe because of a desire to do the best for the patient and society.[62] Factors relating to the wider healthcare system could also be contributing to the possible misuse of antibiotics. In Germany, cost considerations may influence the prescriber. Patients have to pay for weekend call-outs and this was considered as a possible reason for the increase in prescribing on a Friday.[63] This study showed a 23.3% increase in antibiotic prescribing before the weekend. The authors of this study considered that there may have been an increase in the number of patients presenting on Friday with diagnoses that required antibiotics. However, they found that the number of patients presenting with urinary tract infection or respiratory infection was almost the same as on other days of the week. In the UK, patients requiring out-of-hours or weekend treatment are unlikely to be seen by their own GP, so prescribing may occur as a result of the desire to maintain continuity of care. While in the UK weekend care does not have a cost implication, there is perhaps a tendency to prescribe in order that the continuity of care is not compromised. In a study examining the views of diabetic patients regarding their consultations with nurse prescribers, continuity of care was noted as important by almost all of the 41 patients interviewed.[64] The mood of the doctor has also been shown to influence prescribing. A study[65] exploring the association of mood on five behaviours including prescribing found a correlation between negative moods and increased prescribing.

UNCERTAINTY OF DIAGNOSIS AND PROGRESSION OF ILLNESS

Prescribers may be more likely to give a prescription for an antibiotic on a Friday because of the lack of services over the weekend.[66] It may not be clear that a patient requires an antibiotic at the time of consultation but there could be the potential for infection to develop. Prescriptions may be given 'just in case', requiring the patient to make the decision whether to commence treatment. This relies on good information being given at the time of the consultation and the patient understanding both the risks of taking an antibiotic if not necessary and the risks of not taking the antibiotic if the condition becomes worse. In India, patients are known to use their old prescriptions to obtain a new course of antibiotics when experiencing similar conditions that resulted in a prescription for antibiotics previously.[67] This is possible in India as prescriptions are not kept by the pharmacist but given back to patients, which enables reuse. In the UK this would not be possible, as prescriptions are retained by the pharmacist. A lack of understanding by patients of the role of antibiotics can lead to inappropriate prescribing. Prescribers may be pressured to prescribe in circumstances when a patient experiences similar symptoms to those that have previously resulted in a prescription being issued. Some patients may even visit a specific doctor who has previously prescribed. A small study[68] describes instances where nurse practitioners have issued delayed prescriptions despite their better judgement, to 'keep the peace' for children with suspected otitis media, despite guidelines that suggest antibiotics provide little benefit. The risks of antibiotic resistance and the effect on individual patients have been identified through a systematic review.[69] The authors reviewed 24 studies that explored the effect of antibiotic resistance in individuals. They found strong evidence to suggest that those patients who were prescribed an antibiotic for a respiratory or urinary tract infection developed resistance. The resistance was strong in the first month following treatment but could last for up to a year. A 'vicious cycle of resistance' is described, and the authors suggest the way of breaking the cycle is to avoid the prescribing of antibiotics in the first place. By highlighting the effect on individual patients, prescribers may be less likely to consider prescribing an antibiotic where the clinical presentation is uncertain.

LACK OF KNOWLEDGE OR UNDERSTANDING OF THE ROLE OF ANTIBIOTICS

Patients

There is a global need to raise awareness of the role of antibiotics. The United States-based CDC has been running campaigns focused on appropriate antibiotic use since 1995. In 2003 they renamed the campaign 'Get Smart: Know When Antibiotics Work'.[70] The campaign aims to reduce AMR, targeting healthcare providers and the general public by:

- promoting adherence to appropriate prescribing guidelines among providers
- decreasing demand for antibiotics for viral upper respiratory tract infections among healthy adults and parents of young children
- increasing adherence to prescribed antibiotics for upper respiratory tract infections.

The efforts of the CDC are reflected across the globe. The 'Get Smart about Antibiotics' week is supported across the United States by organisations such as the Alliance for the Prudent Use of Antibiotics. In November 2015 the campaign will coincide for the fourth year with similar week-long campaigns in Australia (NPS Medicine Wise), Canada (Antibiotic Awareness) and across Europe (European Antibiotic Awareness Day). The UK is one of 28 European countries participating in the campaign. These campaigns provide online resources for healthcare workers and the public aimed at educating people about the appropriate use of antibiotics. They also provide advice for treating minor ailments such as coughs and colds at home, and explain that in these cases people do not require a visit to the doctor. A range of posters, videos, webinars, factsheets and advice sheets are available from these providers for public and professional use. Campaigns raise awareness of the risks associated with taking antibiotics and how to take them responsibly. They are targeted at the general public, healthcare workers and prescribers in hospital and primary care. Interestingly, in 2009, the UK Department of Health found that, in general, people were confused about bacteria and viruses and what conditions could be treated with antibiotics. The autumn antibiotic campaign was cancelled as a result of this lack of understanding, as well as lack of knowledge in the general public; there was a view that due to the use of antibiotics for secondary infections it may not be the best time to run the campaign, as the public was already confused.[71] It appears there may be little change in public perception of the role of antibiotics since 2009, as more recent qualitative research[72] revealed that of 1767 patients surveyed regarding the use of antibiotics in respiratory infection, 24% of patients believed antibiotics would work for coughs and colds and 38% thought antibiotics would kill viruses. This lack of understanding of the role of antibiotics for certain illnesses has the potential to further increase the misuse of antibiotics. It is possible for the general public across the world to purchase antibiotics over the Internet, although import of prescription-only drugs is illegal in the UK and the United States, and in some countries illegal sale of antibiotics over the counter persists.[73,74] It has been noted[75] that the media, the Internet and other non-credible sources of information are used extensively by patients when searching for information about healthcare-associated infection, which may account for the apparent lack of understanding about the role of antibiotics in infection and the rise of resistant bacteria. Information was viewed as generic with little specific, understandable information available. However, comprehensive advice for patients is available through websites such as NHS Choices[76] and Patient UK[77] in the UK, CDC[78] and the US Department of Health and Human Services Food and Drug Administration[79] in the United States and the European Centre for Disease Prevention and Control,[80] which would seem to address the issue of specificity by providing clear advice aimed at reducing the number of antibiotics prescribed for viral throat infection, for example. Another problem related to understanding that has been identified is that patients may stop taking an antibiotic when they feel better.[81,82] Patients who do not complete a full course of antibiotics could be at risk of prolonged infection and this could contribute to the rise in resistant bacteria.[83]

Prescribers

Not all prescribers themselves are knowledgeable and up to date with current practice guidelines for the use of antibiotics. Numerous guidelines exist for the treatment of infection that are designed to assist the prescriber in their decision that an antibiotic is necessary, but there is evidence to suggest that such guidelines are not always adhered to. In 1998 a report by the UK Standing Medical Advisory Committee[84] stated that many cases of otitis media did not need antibiotics. It was reported later[85] that it was not clear that this had any influence over GP prescribing and that declines in antibiotic prescribing has stabilised since 2000. It has been reported[86] that a similar study undertaken in 2009 showed the continual use of broad-spectrum antibiotics despite guidelines that recommend penicillin V as first choice in acute respiratory tract infection. This study also noted that the higher the number of consultations, the higher the use of antibiotics. In one study[87] designed to explore equality in prescribing across race and insurance status in the United States, it was discovered that despite guidance in 2004 that recommended 'watchful waiting' for acute otitis media, little change in the level of prescribing has been noted, although doctors are using the first-line recommended antibiotic.

It would seem that all health professionals have a role in ensuring the message about the risks of overuse and misuse of antibiotics is clear and consistent. Prescribing of antibiotics should be accompanied with clear instructions and advice about how to take them for the best effect. Prescribing influences should be recognised and acted upon, prescribers must be aware of existing guidance and policy related to antibiotic prescribing, and action to reduce the threat of resistant bacteria should taken. Prudent prescribing requires a multifaceted approach by all healthcare practitioners.

ANTIMICROBIAL STEWARDSHIP

Antimicrobial stewardship aims to reduce inappropriate antibiotic prescribing, therefore reducing the risks of antibiotic-resistant infection and improving outcomes for patients [88] Antimicrobial stewardship is a worldwide initiative for both hospital and outpatient or primary care settings. This initiative is supported in the United States by the 'Get Smart for Health Care' campaign CDC,[89] by the Australian Commission on Safety and Quality in Health Care,[90] and across Europe.[91] and in the UK, 'Start Smart – Then Focus'[92] reminds practitioners of the legal obligation to 'ensure procedures are in place to ensure prudent prescribing and antimicrobial stewardship'. The publication provides clear extensive guidelines for antibiotic prescribing and ongoing management.

The clear message in this document for UK practitioners is only to start antibiotics where a bacterial infection has been clearly identified: once culture has been obtained. Once started, the prescription should be reviewed. Antibiotics should be switched as quickly as possible if necessary when treatment has started prior to cultures being obtained. Intravenous antibiotics should be changed to oral as soon as possible. The programme is focused on use of guidelines, education and audit of practice. Similar guidance is available from the CDC website in the United States. A small study[93] suggests that 'introducing the policy maker' to the decision to prescribe may damage the doctor–patient relationship. The study, while not focused on antibiotic prescribing, found that doctors may wish to preserve the relationship with the patient by using a flexible approach to guidelines. A study undertaken[94] in five European countries and Argentina examined the use of antibiotics in acute exacerbation of chronic obstructive pulmonary disease. The study explored the predictors for prescribing an antibiotic and whether the use of C-reactive protein (CRP) testing reduced prescribing. They found that GPs who used the CRP test were less likely to prescribe an antibiotic. CRP was used as a supplementary test and resulted in fewer antibiotics being prescribed. Tests such as these could be useful in reducing the rate of antibiotic prescribing through clinical presentation alone. Purulent sputum was the highest indicator for a prescription.

There have been calls for all primary care nurses in the UK to be involved in increasing awareness in patient groups of the risks associated with inappropriate antibiotic prescribing.[95] Nurses working in primary care and community are well placed to educate patients about alternatives to antibiotics because nurses were seen as key practitioners, as they spent more time with patients than other healthcare workers.[96] It is indicated that if antimicrobial stewardship programmes are to be successful, they need to take into account the underlying influences that affect prescribing behaviour and not be focused on policy and guidelines.[97] Prescribers want to do the best for patients, to protect them from the harmful effects of infection, to preserve their unique relationships and to ensure practice is responsive to patient need. It is clear that prescribing is a complex process and that many factors influence the decision to prescribe. This is supported by a systematic review[98] undertaken to determine the most effective method of improving antibiotic prescribing in primary care. The review noted that lectures, providing literature and giving feedback did not improve prescribing. Meetings improved prescribing, but it was not clear if visits by educators had any effect. It was noted that the use of delayed prescriptions did decrease antibiotic use. The review concluded that no one intervention was particularly successful on its own but that using different methods together could be successful. Interestingly, a review of the literature relating to interventions for effective antibiotic stewardship in hospitals in 2013[99] revealed that restriction (e.g. needing additional agreement for prescription) and persuasion (e.g. giving feedback or advice on how to prescribe) did improve antibiotic prescribing. The review found that the restrictive methods seemed to have a greater effect.

Much evidence exists to imply that antibiotics are a hindrance in infection control; indeed, it has been stated: 'Control of prescribing would probably be just as effective a measure in our fight against healthcare-associated infection as conventional infection control measures',[100] prescribers need to be supported if we are to 'beat the bugs'. Much more needs to be learned about the factors that influence the decision to prescribe antibiotics; it seems to be clear that there will not be a 'one size fits all' solution.

REFERENCES

1. Department of Health. *UK Five Year Antimicrobial Resistance Strategy 2013 to 2018.* London: Department of Health; 2013. Available at: www.gov.uk/government/uploads/system/uploads/attachment_data/file/244058/20130902_UK_5_year_AMR_strategy.pdf (accessed 20 March 2014).
2. Health and Social Care Information Centre (HSCIC), Prescribing and Primary Care. *Prescription Cost Analysis England 2013.* London: HSCIC; 2012. Available at: www.hscic.gov.uk/article/2021/Website-Search?productid=5461&q=+Prescription+Cost+Analysis+England+2011&sort=Relevance&size=10&page=1&area=both#top (accessed 3 June 2015).
3. Furness H. Resistance to antibiotics could bring 'the end of modern medicine as we know it', WHO claim. *The Telegraph* [online]; 2012 Mar 16. Available at: www.telegraph.co.uk/health/healthnews/9147414/Resistance-to-antibiotics-could-bring-the-end-of-modern-medicine-as-we-know-it-WHO-claim.html (accessed 8 August 2012).
4. Ledwith M. Why a sore throat could soon be fatal: Bugs are becoming more resistant to antibiotics, warn health chiefs. *Mail Online* [online]; 2012. Available at: www.dailymail.co.uk/news/article-2115722/Why-sore-throat-soon-fatal-Bugs-resistant-antibiotics-warn-health-chiefs.html (accessed 8 August 2012).
5. European Commission. *Communication from the Commission to the European Parliament and the Council: action plan against the rising threats from antimicrobial resistance.* Communication 2011/748/EC. Brussels: European Commission; 2011.
6. Health Protection Agency. *Over Half of All People Who Visit their Doctor with Coughs and Colds Still Expect Antibiotics.* London: Health Protection Agency; 2011. Available at: www.hpa.org.uk/NewsCentre/NationalPressReleases/2011PressReleases/111118Antibioticawarenessday/ (accessed 29 July 2012).
7. World Health Organization (WHO). *The Evolving Threat of Antimicrobial Resistance: options for action.* Geneva: WHO; 2012.
8. WHO, op. cit.
9. Standing Medical Advisory Committee Sub-Group on Antimicrobial Resistance. *The Path of Least Resistance.* London: Department of Health; 1998.
10. Department of Health, op. cit.
11. Davies S, Gibbens N. *UK Five Year Antimicrobial Resistance Strategy 2013 to 2018.* London: Department of Health; 2013.
12. Joint Formulary Committee. *British National Formulary.* 67th ed. London: BMJ Group and Pharmaceutical Press; 2014.
13. Nathwani D, Morgan M, Masterton RG, et al. British Society for Antimicrobial Chemotherapy Working Party on Community-onset MRSA Infections. Guidelines for UK practice for the diagnosis and management of methicillin-resistant *Staphylococcus aureus* (MRSA) infections presenting in the community. *J Antimicrob Chemother.* 2008; **61**(5): 976–94.
14. Department of Health, op. cit.
15. Paterson DL, Bonomo RA. Extended-spectrum β-lactamases: a clinical update. *Clin Microbiol Rev.* 2005; **18**(4): 657–86.
16. Joint Formulary Committee, op. cit.
17. Public Health England. *Acute Trust Toolkit for the Early Detection, Management and Control of Carbapenemase-Producing Enterobacteriaceae.* London: Public Health England; 2013.
18. Public Health England, op. cit.
19. Public Health England, op. cit.
20. Public Health England, op. cit.

21. WHO, op. cit.
22. WHO, op. cit.
23. European Commission, op. cit.
24. WHO, op. cit.
25. WHO, op. cit.
26. Department of Health, op. cit.
27. Medicine and Healthcare Products Regulatory Agency. Tigecycline (Tygacil): increased mortality in clinical trials – use only when other antibiotics are unsuitable. *Drug Safety Update*. 2011; 4 April. Available at: www.gov.uk/drug-safety-update/tigecycline-tygacil-increased-mortality-in-clinical-trials (accessed 25 June 2015).
28. Department of Health, op. cit.
29. Department of Health, op. cit.
30. WHO, op. cit.
31. WHO, op. cit.
32. Centers for Disease Control and Prevention. *Antibiotic Resistance Threats in the United States, 2013*. US Department of Health and Human Services; 2013.
33. Currie J, Lin W, Zhang W. Patient knowledge and antibiotic abuse: evidence from an audit study in China. *J Health Econ*. 2011; **30**: 933–49.
34. Costelloe C, Metcalfe C, Lovering A, *et al*. Effect of antibiotic prescribing in primary care on antimicrobial resistance in individual patients: systematic review and meta-analysis. *BMJ*. 2010; **340**: c2096. Available at: www.bmj.com/content/340/bmj.c2096 (accessed 11 August 2012).
35. Public Health England, op. cit.
36. Finch R, Metlay J, Davey P, *et al*. Educational interventions to improve antibiotic use in the community: report from the International Forum on Antibiotic Resistance (IFAR) colloquium, 2002 Antibiotic Resistance colloquium (2002). *Lancet Infect Dis*. 2004; **4**(1): 44–53. Erratum in: *Lancet Infect Dis*. 2004; **4**(3): 185.
37. World Health Organization (WHO). *Antimicrobial Resistance: factsheet No. 194*. Geneva: WHO; 2013. Available at: www.who.int/mediacentre/factsheets/fs194/en/ (accessed 14 October 2013).
38. Costelloe, *et al*., op. cit.
39. Vazquez-Lago J, Lopez-Vazquez P, López-Durán A, *et al*. Attitudes of primary care physicians to the prescribing of antibiotics and antimicrobial resistance: a qualitative study from Spain. *Fam Pract*. 2012; **29**(3): 352–60.
40. Rodrigues A, Roquea F, Falcãob A, *et al*. Understanding physician antibiotic prescribing behaviour: a systematic review of qualitative studies. *Int J Antimicrob Agents*. 2013; **41**(3): 203–12.
41. Kotwania A, Wattal C, Katewa S, *et al*. Factors influencing primary care physicians to prescribe antibiotics in Delhi India. *Fam Pract*. 2010; **27**(6): 684–90.
42. Kuehlein T, Szecsenyi J, Gutscher A, *et al*. Antibiotic prescribing in general practice – the rhythm of the week: a cross-sectional study. *J Antimicrob Chemother*. 2010; **65**(12): 2666–8.
43. Hajjaj M, Salek M, Basra M, *et al*. Non-clinical influences on clinical decision making: a major challenge to evidence-based practice. *J Royal Soc Med*. 2010; **103**(5): 178–87.
44. Philp A, Winfield L. Why prescribe antibiotics for otitis media in children? *Nurs Prescribing*. 2010; **8**(1): 14–19.
45. Wood F, Simpson S, Butler C. Socially responsible antibiotic choices in primary care: a qualitative study of GPs' decisions to prescribe broad-spectrum and fluoroquinolone antibiotics. *Fam Pract*. 2007; **24**(5): 427–34.

46. Lopez-Vazquez P, Juan M, Vazquez-Lago M, *et al*. Misprescription of antibiotics in primary care: a critical systematic review of its determinants. *J Eval Clin Pract*. 2012; **18**(2): 473–84.

47. Brookes-Howell L, Hood K, Cooper L, *et al*. Understanding variation in primary medical care: a nine-country qualitative study of clinicians' accounts of the non-clinical factors that shape antibiotic prescribing decisions for lower respiratory tract infection. *BMJ Open*. 2012; **22**(4): e000796. Available at: http://bmjopen.bmj.com/content/2/4/e000796.full.pdf+html (accessed 2 January 2014).

48. Vazquez-Lago, *et al*., op. cit.

49. Hajjaj, *et al*., op. cit.

50. Hulscher M, Meer J, Grol R. Antibiotic use: how to improve it? *Int J Med Microbiol*. 2010; **300**(6): 351–6.

51. Kotwania, op. cit.

52. Philp, Winfield, op. cit.

53. Wood, Simpson, Butler, op. cit.

54. Scoggins A, Tiessen J, Ling T, *et al*. *Prescribing in Primary Care: understanding what shapes GPs' prescribing choices and how might these be changed*. Cambridge: RAND Corporation; 2006.

55. Grant A, Sullivan F, Dowell J. An ethnographic exploration of influences on prescribing in general practice: why is there variation in prescribing practices? *Implementation Sci*. 2013; **8**(72). Available at: www.implementationscience.com/content/8/1/72 (accessed 19 December 2013).

56. World Health Organization. *Worldwide Country Situation Analysis: response to antimicrobial resistance*. Geneva: World Health Organization; 2015.

57. Finch, *et al*., op. cit.

58. Arnold SR, Straus SE. Interventions to improve antibiotic prescribing practices in ambulatory care. *Cochrane Database Syst Rev*. 2009; (4): CD003539.

59. Hulscher, Meer, Grol, op. cit.

60. Philp, Winfield, op. cit.

61. ProCon.org. *Prescription Drug Ads. Should prescription drugs be advertised direct to consumers?* ProCon.org; 2014. Available at: http://prescriptiondrugs.procon.org/ (accessed 4 June 2015).

62. Wood, Simpson, Butler, op. cit.

63. Kuehlein, *et al*., op. cit.

64. Stenner K, Courtenay M, Carey N. Consultations between nurse prescribers and patients with diabetes in primary care: a qualitative study of patient views. *Int J Nurs Stud*. 2011; **48**(1): 37–46.

65. Kushnir T, Kushnir J, Sarelc A, *et al*. Exploring physician perceptions of the impact of emotions on behaviour during interactions with patients. *Fam Pract*. 2011; **28**: 75–8.

66. Botica M, Botica I, Stameni V, *et al*. Antibiotic prescription rate for upper respiratory tract infections and risks for unnecessary prescription in Croatia. *Coll Antropol*. 2013; **37**(2): 449–54. Available at: http://hrcak.srce.hr/index.php?show=clanak&id_clanak_jezik=153603&lang=en (accessed 2 January 2014).

67. Kotwania, op. cit.

68. Philp, Winfield, op. cit.

69. Costelloe, *et al*., op. cit.

70. Centers for Disease Control and Prevention. 2015. *Get Smart: Know When Antibiotics Work*. Available at www.cdc.gov/getsmart/community/index.html (accessed 29 July 2015).

71. Moberly T. Antibiotic campaign scrapped over 'confusion' – News. *Independent Nurse.* 2009 Nov 20: 3.

72. McNulty C, Nichols T, French DP, *et al.* Expectations for consultations and antibiotics for respiratory tract infection in primary care: the RTI clinical iceberg. *Br J Gen Pract.* 2013; **63**(612): e429–36. Available at: http://bjgp.org/content/63/612/e429.full.pdf+html (accessed 2 January 2014).

73. Llor C, Cots JM. The sale of antibiotics without prescription in pharmacies in Catalonia, Spain. *Clin Infect Dis.* 2009; **48**(10): 1345–9.

74. Al-Faham Z, Habboub G, Takriti F. The sale of antibiotics without prescription in pharmacies in Damascus, Syria. *J Infect Dev Ctries.* 2011; **5**(5): 396–9. Available at: http://jidc.org/index.php/journal/article/viewFile/1248/553 (accessed 2 January 2014).

75. Gould D, Drey NS, Millar M, *et al.* Patients and the public: knowledge, sources of information and perceptions about healthcare associated infection. *J Hosp Infect.* 2009; **72**(1): 1–8.

76. NHS Choices. *Sore Throat.* Available at: www.nhs.uk/conditions/sore-throat/pages/introduction.aspx (accessed 4 June 2015).

77. Patient UK. *Antibiotics.* Available at: http://patient.info/health/antibiotics-leaflet (accessed 4 June 2015).

78. Centers for Disease Control and Prevention. 2013. Available at: www.cdc.gov/getsmart/community/for-patients/common-illnesses/sore-throat.html (accessed 4 June 2015).

79. US Department of Health and Human Services Food and Drug Administration. *Preserve a Treasure: know when antibiotics work.* Available at: www.fda.gov/downloads/Drugs/ResourcesForYou/UCM233219.pdf (accessed 4 June 2015).

80. European Centre for Disease Prevention and Control (ECDC). *Streptococcal Pharyngitis:* factsheet for the general public. Sweden: ECDC; 2013. Available at: www.ecdc.europa.eu/en/healthtopics/streptococcal_pharyngitis/pages/factsheet_general_public.aspx (accessed 10 December 2013).

81. Hawkings N, Butler C, Wood F. Antibiotics in the community: a typology of user behaviours. *Patient Educ Couns.* 2008; **73**(1): 146–52.

82. Chan YC, Fan M, Fok CM, *et al.* Antibiotics nonadherence and knowledge in a community with the world's leading prevalence of antibiotics resistance: Implications for public health intervention. *Am J Infect Control.* 2012; **40**(2): 113–17.

83. Patient UK. *Sore Throat.* Available at: http://patient.info/health/sore-throat-leaflet (accessed 4 June 2015).

84. Standing Medical Advisory Committee Sub-Group on Antimicrobial Resistance. *The Path of Least Resistance.* London: Department of Health; 1998.

85. Thompson P, Gilbert R, Long P, *et al.* Has UK guidance affected general practitioner antibiotic prescribing for otitis media in children? *J Pub Health.* 2008; **30**(4): 479–86.

86. Gjelstad S, Straand J, Dalen I, *et al.* Do general practitioners' consultation rates influence their prescribing patterns of antibiotics for acute respiratory tract infections? *J Antimicrob Chemother.* 2011; **66**(10): 2425–33.

87. Sidell D, Shapiro NL, Bhattacharyya N. Demographic influences on antibiotic prescribing for pediatric acute otitis media. *Otolaryngol Head Neck Surg.* 2012; **146**(4): 653–8.

88. Ashiru-Oredope D, Sharland M, Charani E, *et al.* Improving the quality of antibiotic prescribing in the NHS by developing a new antimicrobial stewardship programme: Start Smart – Then Focus. *J Antimicrob Chemother.* 2012; **67**(Suppl. 1): S51–63.

89. Centers for Disease Control and Prevention. *Implementing and Improving Stewardship Efforts.* Available at: www.cdc.gov/getsmart/healthcare/improve-efforts/index.html (accessed 4 June 2015).

90. Australian Commission on Safety and Quality in Health Care. *Antimicrobial Stewardship Initiative*. Available at: www.safetyandquality.gov.au/our-work/healthcare-associated-infection/antimicrobial-stewardship/ (accessed 4 June 2015).

91. Allerberger F, Gareis R, Jindrák V, *et al.* Antibiotic stewardship implementation in the EU: the way forward. *Expert Rev Anti Infect Ther.* 2009; **7**(10): 1175–83. Available at: http://informahealthcare.com/doi/pdf/10.1586/eri.09.96 (accessed 2 January 2014).

92. Department of Health. *Antimicrobial Stewardship: Start Smart – Then Focus.* Available at: www.gov.uk/government/publications/antimicrobial-stewardship-start-smart-then-focus (accessed 2 January 2014).

93. Solomon J, Raynor DK, Knapp P, *et al.* The compatibility of prescribing guidelines and the doctor–patient partnership: a primary care mixed-methods study. *Br J Gen Pract.* 2012; **62**(597): e275-81. doi: 10.3399/bjgp12X636119.

94. Llor C, Bjerrum L, Munck A, *et al.* Predictors for antibiotic prescribing in patients with exacerbations of COPD in general practice. *Ther Adv Respir Dis.* 2013; **7**(3): 131–7.

95. Lepper J. Nurses urged to lead awareness drive about risks of antibiotics. *Independent Nurse.* 2011 Nov 21: 5.

96. Gillespie E, Rodrigues A, Wright L, *et al.* Improving antibiotic stewardship by involving nurses. *Am J Infect Control.* 2013; **41**(4): 365–7.

97. Charani E, Cooke J, Holmes A. Antibiotic stewardship programmes – what's missing? *J Antimicrob Chemother.* 2013; **65**: 2275–7.

98. Arnold, Strauss, op. cit.

99. Davey P, Brown E, Charani E, *et al.* Interventions to improve antibiotic prescribing practices for hospital inpatients. *Cochrane Database Syst Rev.* 2013; (4): CD003543.

100. Gould IM. Controversies in infection: infection control or antibiotic stewardship to control healthcare-acquired infection? *J Hosp Infec.* 2009; **73**(4): e386–91.

CHAPTER 9

The impact of *Clostridium difficile* infection on patients and their families

....

Graziella Kontkowski

In July 2005, shortly after arriving for Sunday lunch with my family, my grandmother was admitted to hospital. She was taken by ambulance to the nearest accident and emergency, where she was examined and blood and urine samples were taken. I was informed that it seemed she was suffering from a severe urinary tract infection and that she was required to be admitted for intravenous antibiotics. Granny responded well to the treatment, but after about 5 days of being in hospital she suffered a setback – she had developed a further infection (osteomyelitis), which was to delay her discharge.

I was visiting her in hospital every day, and on first impressions the ward looked like any other ward providing care of the elderly. There were five beds to each bay. Two of the beds opposite my Granny were occupied; one of these women never seemed to have any visitors and the other had a constant stream of visitors who were present with her most of the time. One of the things that I do clearly remember about one of these women was the smell that travelled through the bay after she opened her bowels: it was foul and offensive, and being July the temperature was too high, which didn't help the situation. I noticed more and more people were coming to see her and I soon realised that this was because she had become very unwell. Sadly, she died. At the time, I didn't know what caused her death; little did I know I was soon to find out.

During one of my evening visits I was greeted by a nurse who informed me that my Gran had 'a little bug'. I didn't think too much about it – I knew tummy bugs lasted a couple of days, so I wasn't too worried. A couple of days passed but Granny wasn't getting any better; in fact, she looked worse. At this stage I was informed that she would have to be put into one of the isolation rooms. I asked questions but no one was telling me what was wrong. I was promised some information and, in passing, one of the senior house officers told me that the bug Granny was suffering from was *Clostridium difficile*. Granny was now experiencing constant diarrhoea. It was relentless; she could not control her bowels and she often had accidents in the bed while waiting for the bed pan to be brought to her. She started to suffer from bed sores. She had no appetite and would only drink when someone pushed her to, resulting in her becoming dehydrated and then her kidneys began to fail. How on earth was this happening? Why was no one ensuring that she was drinking when I wasn't with her to do this?

There were so many things that worried me about her care, with the casual approach of the nursing staff being number one on my list. In fact, there were one or two nurses who really should not have been working in a profession that is supposed to care for others, because there was nothing about them that conveyed to me that they cared about their patients. I found tablets on the floor – tablets that were supposed to be given to my Granny; soiled linen left in a corner of her room time and time again; dirty bed pans being brought in for her to sit on; and on one occasion I found her intravenous line hanging out of her arm with the pump still pushing fluids through, resulting in the floor being covered with saline, the list went on and on. I was disgusted and upset that in this day and age I was witnessing such a poor standard of care here in the United Kingdom.

The environmental cleaning was another issue that concerned me greatly. While there were cleaners who would come in to clean the room, most of the time they looked half asleep. I witnessed them give the room a very superficial clean – the dust was so thick in places it could have made a blanket. The curtains were dirty and there were visible stains on the walls. It was clear that these staff were not fulfilling their basic duties. I felt helpless and I didn't know what to do. I was so unhappy about leaving my Granny in this environment but I felt there was very little I could do. I couldn't bring her home, because she was too unwell, but I couldn't just sit back and watch what was happening on the ward. Like many relatives who have to leave their loved ones in the care of healthcare staff, I was at a loss: I didn't know what to do. I considered complaining but I was anxious that Granny was vulnerable and completely dependent on the staff to care for her; however, I decided I had no alternative. I had to complain. This wasn't just for my Granny: this was for other patients too, other patients who had no one to speak up for them.

What staff have to remember is that the patients they look after are someone's mother, father, brother, sister, son or daughter and in my case my grandmother. They are in hospital because they have to be, because they are ill. Often they are very vulnerable and frightened being in an environment that is alien to them. Therefore, it is important that staff do their utmost to ensure that the patients they care for are always treated with the dignity and respect they deserve. One final thing to remember is that, one day, that patient could be one of your own loved ones or perhaps even yourself; therefore, never give care that you yourself would not be prepared to accept.

My dear Granny wasn't doing well at all. She had become a shadow of her former self. This larger-than-life Italian woman was now transformed into a very frail, very sick old lady who was going to die from an infection she contracted in hospital on a dirty ward with uncaring staff. It broke my heart watching her. I felt so guilty – guilty about so many things. Why did I allow the ambulance to take her to this particular hospital, the hospital where my mother had died at the age of 49 from complications of cholecystitis, and where we hadn't set foot for the 15 years that had followed? I felt guilty about not being able to be with her as much as I wanted to. I felt guilty that I couldn't do more to alleviate her suffering, and I felt guilty that it took me so long to speak up, something that I should never have had to do if the care she was given were of a good standard.

After my complaint, Granny was moved back onto the open ward because it was now being used as a cohort ward, with 30 patients infected with *C. difficile*. I felt that at least she would not be as neglected on the open ward as she had been in the isolation room, but how wrong I was. It made no difference, because the staff on the ward could not to cope with such a huge outbreak. It was complete chaos. Staff could not keep up with the volume of patients suffering with diarrhoea; the smell on the ward is something that I will never forget.

It was such a distressing time for me: my Granny had been a huge part of my life for so long and now I was watching her die and I felt I could do nothing to help her. You may say that she was 93, that she had lived her life, that we all have to go one day – and of course we do – but it was watching her suffer in the way she did that was heartbreaking and which left me feeling helpless.

In September I went in to visit her and at this time I knew that Granny had lost her fight. The look on her face as she saw me approaching the bed is an image that I will never forget. She held her hand out to me and tried to speak, yet words were not coming out. She looked so frightened. There were nurses in the bay but they did not seem to see how distressed she was. Her hands were so cold, she looked pale and her body was shutting down, yet nobody seemed to be doing anything. I asked the nurses to get a doctor to come to see her. In my heart I knew that she was dying, but I still wanted someone to tell me she would be OK. The doctor came but she didn't do very much: she had a quick look at Granny and spoke about giving her some fluids, but I could see it was now just a matter of time. I called my brother to join me at the hospital. I made arrangements for my children to be looked after and, between my brother and I, we sat with her day and night until she took her last breath at 4.30 p.m. on Monday 26 September 2005.

Yes, my grandmother was old and had lived a full life, but no one should have to go through what she went through, and die in the way she did, with a lack of dignity and compassion. So many illnesses that were once a death sentence are now treatable. We have so many technologies and new methods in many parts of healthcare to detect problems before they happen, yet here I witnessed a preventable infection kill someone I loved. I constantly search for answers to the question: 'Were there things that could have prevented my grandmother from contracting C. difficile?' I know now that the answer to this question is yes, and I feel the overuse of antibiotics has played a major part in the explosion of these lethal infections. However, in my grandmother's case she needed antibiotics to treat what was fast becoming a life-threatening sepsis. While antibiotics may have played a part in my grandmother's condition, I firmly believe that a lack of basic hygiene was also a major factor. It seemed that no one at the hospital was taking the problem seriously until it was too late, and by this time the infection was rampant on the ward. Simple things such as good hand hygiene and careful environmental cleaning could have helped to prevent infection for not only my grandmother but also many other patients. This outbreak of C. difficile contributed to a very tough workload for staff. My grandmother was not mobile, so it is highly likely that the infection had been passed on to her from the hands of a healthcare professional, something that could have been avoided if staff had taken the time to wash their hands. Something so simple could have prevented the spread of this lethal infection.

Since 2005 there have been many improvements in infection prevention and control and the numbers of infections have been falling. However, I would urge all healthcare professionals to think over my words as they provide their care and treatment to vulnerable patients, and in particular to remember to always do the right thing: cleaning your hands at the right time and making sure wards are clean and safe. Always remember to follow your infection control protocols, because I am sure no one would want to be responsible for passing an avoidable infection to a patient.

Something as simple as cleaning your hands can make a big difference to the outcome of your patient's care; therefore, I would urge everyone who cares for patients to never become complacent and to never think that hand hygiene can be overlooked because 'there isn't time'. Washing your hands takes less than a minute, so never say, 'I haven't got time'. Not only will that minute save you time – time having to look after someone suffering from an avoidable infection – but also, and more important, that minute really can save lives.

CHAPTER 10

The challenge we all face together

Derek Butler

In being asked to contribute a chapter for this book I asked myself, what could I contribute that would make an impact and enlighten those of you in healthcare who care for others, especially in respect to healthcare-associated infections? Although I am not a healthcare professional, I have been affected by events surrounding healthcare infections that could primarily have been avoided.

As you will have already seen in this book, there are many contributions from eminent people in the healthcare profession and patient groups looking at reasons why and how we can ensure patients receive clean, safe care, free from the fear of contracting an avoidable healthcare infection. The effect such an infection has on pain, suffering and loss of dignity; on patients and their families, is all too apparent. When the system fails it has a ripple effect that leaves an unwanted legacy.

However, for my own contribution, I would like to dedicate this chapter to the memory of the most important people concerned within this book: the patients who have suffered, and their loved ones who lost someone to an avoidable healthcare infection. I would like to dedicate this chapter especially to my dear friend and stepfather, John Crews, whom our family tragically lost at the age of 54. I would also like to dedicate this chapter to those families who have lost loved ones and with whom I have met. These include the families of people such as Sue Fallon, who lost her daughter at the age of 17 and who had to tell her youngest daughter that her sister would not be coming home from hospital; Paul Kelly, who lost his pregnant daughter Clare at the age of 23 and his unborn grandson; Mavis Law, whose son Colin died the day before his 33rd birthday when admitted to hospital for tests; 68-year-old Patricia Galvin, who bravely fought cancer only to succumb to meticillin-resistant *Staphylococcus aureus* (MRSA); and Patricia Lloyd, a mother who contracted MRSA and died after treatment from a community dentist. In addition, the many other families I have come into contact with as chair of MRSA Action UK.

Probably the hardest thing anyone can experience is to lose a loved one. I have experienced first-hand the effects healthcare-associated infections have on those who contract them and on the family left behind. Certainly, in life I have learned there are certain events that shape a person's life. For me, having my stepfather in my life helped to develop whom I am today; however, the event that shaped the life I have now, and which was the hardest thing I have ever done, was to hold my stepfather in my arms and watch him die. This was a man who was the greatest influence in my life, a man whom I called my friend, a person whom I could rely on to turn to for help if I needed to. My stepfather was a man who had helped me all my life, yet at the moment he passed away I felt helpless in not being able to prevent his death. However, the aspect of this event that shaped my life the most was that even at the time my stepfather died, we were never informed that he was profusely infected with MRSA, despite the staff and the hospital knowing this for 7 days before his death. Once we discovered the facts and that the staff and hospital knew of the infections, like all the families I have mentioned, we determined ourselves to prevent this from happening again to other families.

I questioned myself, how could anyone be lost to an infection in the twenty-first century with all the modern healthcare facilities, with all the modern drugs especially antibiotics, the golden bullets and all the knowledge mankind has accumulated in combating bacteria? With the help of others, MRSA Action UK was born to seek answers to our questions. I want to look at this from a more personal perspective and perception for us all, for future generations and all our families. I would like to make this thought-provoking and challenging and, more important, I would like to look to the long view on why it is vital to control bacteria in our medical and community facilities, and why the loss of the efficacy of antibiotics will have an impact on all our futures.

Let us remember that the majority of people alive or reading this chapter today were born in an antibiotic era. If you get an infection today, the answer is simple: just take an antibiotic. For how much longer will this be the answer? It would be wise for us to remember that within living memory it was not always like this. In the early to the middle part of the twentieth century, over 50% of people did not live past the age of 65. Infection was the leading cause of death and people used to live in mortal fear of bacterial infections. There was no cure; the only defence was scrupulous hygiene, both in the home and in hospital. Antibiotics changed all of that, and their discovery gave mankind the greatest leap in medical science it had ever known, opening new avenues to treatments once thought impossible.

Imagine what it must have been like in our hospitals in the early part of the twentieth century, in respect to infection prevention and control before the discovery of antibiotics. Hygiene and cleanliness was far more stringent then than it is at present. Ask yourself honestly, could you and your colleagues manage to perform your duties today as your predecessors did all those years ago but without the current-day advantages you have, advantages that they could never have dreamed of?

Why is it so important to have effective infection prevention and control systems that leave no gaps for bacteria to infect patients or enter our hospitals and the community? Let us be under no illusions as to the importance of good infection prevention and control and what this means to us, to future generations and, moreover, to the future of modern medicine. Our failure to take the correct action necessary now will place the future of modern medicine, as we know it, in jeopardy. Our failure in infection prevention and control will add pressure to our dwindling stocks of antibiotics, leaving the possibility that resistant bacteria will become dominant and leaving modern healthcare medicine as we know it consigned to the history books.

This would mean medical procedures that were only dreamed of less than 40 years ago but which we now take for granted would become non-existent. This would in effect make our healthcare system return to a position not seen by our generation or even our parents' generation. Therefore, it is in our own interests to ensure that we as parents pass on to our children a healthcare system far better than the one we inherited from our own parents.

Where does infection control fit into all of this? You as infection control staff have the skills, knowledge, ability and responsibility to alter what many think is inevitable. If you talk to the families who have lost a loved one to what is, for all intents and purposes, an avoidable healthcare infection, they will tell you that it leaves a legacy that cannot be erased. They will tell you it leaves a legacy of helplessness and of bewilderment that their loved one has died from something that not that long ago was treatable with a positive outcome. They then look to the past with puzzlement as to how we managed to find ourselves in this situation, and they fear for the future of their children and grandchildren and whether they will receive the medical care we take for granted.

Those same families and individuals have said to me, do the medical staff not realise that our concerns are their concerns, our children and grandchildren are their children and grandchildren, and it is their future healthcare we are putting at risk when we ignore this problem? They ask me, do the staff have no concerns that while we erode the use of these magic bullets called antibiotics, we are consigning future generations to a life that will be far worse than the one we have lived?

Therefore, what can be done to try to reverse this situation? Well, you as healthcare professionals are in the unique position of being able to slow down this problem of contracting avoidable healthcare infections by your own actions and thoughts. You do not have to accept that some things are inevitable: they are not, otherwise we would not have progressed to the point where we are as a species today. We have progressed because we challenge, we do not accept the inevitable and we change the norm.

A great American leader once said, 'If you are aware something is wrong, if you have the ability to correct that wrong, then you have placed upon you the responsibility to correct that wrong' (Anon). We are all in a battle against the formidable enemy that is bacteria, an enemy that can mutate and change and spread with impunity. However, the Achilles heel of bacteria is that many cannot survive in their own environment and rely on the conditions created by humans. However, if those conditions are changed and controlled then bacteria will find it very difficult to cause harm both now and in the future. What words of advice can I give you, a person who represents those who have been affected by avoidable healthcare infection and one who has seen the effect this has had on my family first-hand?

It doesn't matter how efficiently the hospital functions; how good the training, supervision and procedures are; or how well the best worker, doctor, nurse, cleaner or manager performs his or her duties. People cannot perform better than the organisation supporting them; so ensure that you and your colleagues change the system to support you, because you don't just want to succeed, you also want to excel. While 'success' means being the best, 'excellence' means being *at your best*. The quality of excelling is an ongoing pursuit to continually ensure that you can give your patients and their families the confidence that everything that can be done to ensure their safety is being done.

The greatest tribute you can give, in memory of those who have suffered and been lost to avoidable healthcare infections, is to do all that you can, in spite of all the difficulties you face, to ensure that no patient contracts an avoidable infection on your watch. I hope that when you have finished reading this book, you will ask yourself and your colleagues one simple question: What are we going to do differently when we go back to care for our patients that we are not doing now?

I would like to finish with a few thoughts from our organisation, MRSA Action UK. Our organisation was born out of the pain we felt at losing a loved one to an avoidable healthcare infection. However, we must remember that in the final analysis our most common basic link is that we will all use the same healthcare system. We all want safe, clean care, and we all cherish our children's future and want them to receive the same safe, clean care, but we should also remember that we are all mortal.

My final thought comes from Edmund Burke,[1] who said:

> All that is necessary for the triumph of evil is that good men do nothing.

Let us change this to:

> All that is necessary for the triumph of bacteria is that good people do nothing.

We, the staff in the National Health Service, the patients, their families and patient support groups such as MRSA Action UK must work together on this, in the memory of those who have been lost. Failure to do so will leave a legacy for our children and grandchildren that they will never forgive us for. Let us not throw away the legacy Sir Alexander Fleming gave us regarding antibiotics, and let us always bear in mind importance of doing the right thing, first time every time in combating resistant bacteria.

REFERENCE

1. The Quotations Page. *Quotations by Author: Edmund Burke (1729–1797)*. QuotationsPage. com. Available at: www.quotationspage.com/quotes/Edmund_Burke/ (accessed 9 January 2015).

PART III

Possibilities for infection prevention and control

No stone left unturned: the relevance of the neurosciences to infection prevention and control

....

Julie Storr

We have mapped the human genome but we still cannot get healthcare workers to clean their hands at the right time.

It weighs roughly the same as a bag of self-raising flour, is made largely of fat and water, and is the target of most of what we do in infection prevention and control (IPC). And right now, it's sitting inside your head as you read this book. The brain. The organ that controls everything we do, how we think and perceive the world around us and, importantly, how we behave. For those of us interested in improving practice it is critical that we understand the determinants of behaviour. Such an understanding offers much in relation to getting and keeping people's attention, getting inside another person's mind, to influence behaviours, to change or instil habits, to stimulate a person to do something that will make or keep that person safe. A full understanding will only enhance the impact of the policies we write, the training we provide, the social interactions, the advice on the telephone, our communication. This chapter will pose a series of questions designed to stimulate those interested in IPC, to consider some of the available disciplines and what they have to offer in our quest to get better at influencing and changing behaviour in the pursuit of saving lives.

My first question, one that has niggled away at me for some years is: why is there such a position of behavioural epidemiologist but not yet one of behavioural IPC nurse or doctor – what does the answer to this question tell us? That there is no such position suggests that we may need to move a little faster in order to fully integrate the behavioural and the social sciences within the specialty. In 2012, a systematic review by Edwards and colleagues[1] found that theoretical frameworks from psychology, social marketing and other social sciences that address the issue of how to change behaviour and sustain changes over time are widely underused in IPC. Elliott[2] did much to introduce the concept of the psychosocial aspects of infection control through his book of 2009, and it's fitting to mention the *WHO Guidelines on Hand Hygiene in Health Care*,[3] which devoted an entire chapter to behaviour change. The multimodal strategy that falls out of these guidelines promotes this strategy as the ultimate 'bundle' for improvement. The multimodal strategy is constructed around a number of theories of behaviour change, drawing on work relating to motivation from the 1980s and 1990s when colleagues introduced us to the Theory of Planned Behaviour[4] and the Health Belief Model[5] as applied to hand hygiene improvement. In the early days of infection prevention, and potentially even today, most of what academics describe often seems disconnected to the day-to-day activities of IPC.

Let's quickly summarise the essence of IPC. It is an evidence-based multidisciplinary specialty that is concerned with putting in place important processes and interventions that affect patient outcomes. Through surveillance and feedback of data, IPC practitioners should provide the necessary data to drive action and alert the organisation to potential outbreaks. Through education and training programmes, IPC endeavours to provide the requisite knowledge for safe practice, whether that be about organisational or local guidelines related to the insertion and maintenance of a urinary catheter or the utilisation and control of antibiotics. Ultimately, it exists to reassure patients and the public that healthcare workers practise in a way that maximises safety and minimises harm. Much of IPC, therefore, is concerned with implementation of established best practice guidance. Implementation is about the way people behave. Facilitating the desired behaviour relies on a combination of methods, not solely a technical understanding of clinical microbiology. It is on implementation and behaviour change that this chapter will now focus.

Recently, Michie and colleagues[6] have distilled 19 theories of behaviour change and packaged them within the progressive and excellent Behaviour Change Wheel. The Behaviour Change Wheel acts as a fulcrum on which to propose that there remain as yet unexplored approaches within the social sciences that may contain additional sources of strength to help us influence change. In fact, I will go deeper to consider how the world of neuroscience, neurolinguistic programming (NLP) and hypnotherapy might present some insights that could at least add value to current approaches. Within the context of motivation, this chapter poses a question to the infection prevention community: in the quest for impact, has enough attention been paid to these fields and their possible utility? Do they have something or nothing to offer us in the twenty-first century?

WHAT CAN WE LEARN FROM THE BEHAVIOURAL SCIENCES?

The Behaviour Change Wheel provides a framework for developing interventions that addresses the different influencers and determinants of behaviour and is increasingly being used in public health and infection prevention. It acts as a guide to securing the right behaviour change techniques in a certain context. It addresses the interventions that are developed to change behaviour and the policies that promote or support them. At its heart it addresses capability, motivation and opportunity as the sources of behaviour that we need to fully analyse in order to have the right influence at the policy and political level.

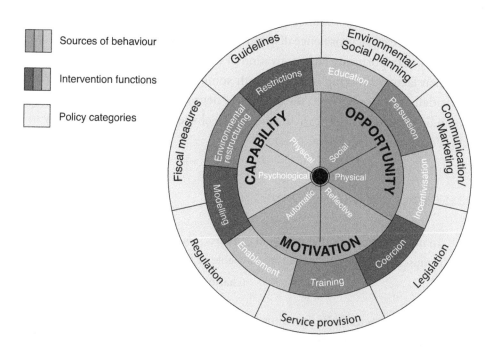

FIGURE 11.1 The Behaviour Change Wheel (reproduced with permission of BioMed Central from Michie *et al.*[6])

A recent RSA (Royal Society for the encouragement of Arts, Manufactures and Commerce) report[7] reminds us that in order to be clear about the different approaches to behaviour change it is necessary to understand the two systems of the human brain, the controlled system and the automatic system. The former is concerned with thinking, goal seeking and deliberate actions, while the latter is more intuitive and instinctive. Appreciation of these two systems and attempts to exploit them is the basis for much of what is termed behavioural economics and nudge theory.[8] Daniel Kahneman's[9] fascinating book provides many insights into how the two systems work and why we need to understand these in a behaviour change context. Nudge theory is an extension of behavioural economics and attempts to influence behaviour through developing social policies informed by neuroscience and psychology. Application of nudge theory has led to adjusting the language and simplifying messages used in formal communications to encourage people to comply, for example, with outstanding debts. There are many examples of this being successful, although it is not without its critics. Nudge theory is also being applied in the field of public health, where, for example, changes to the environment such as designing buildings with fewer lifts encourage people to expend energy walking up stairs. Building on these examples, to what extent can some of the not-so-mainstream neuroscience disciplines help influence behaviour by affecting the capability, opportunity and motivation of our target audience?

Human factors thinking is aligned with some of the ideas of nudge theory. It is potentially a bridge between the concept of neuroscience and the reality of how this can be applied in healthcare to address the challenges of practising safely in a highly complex sociotechnical system.[10]

DISSECTING THE BRAIN: CONNECTOMES

> To move things is all that mankind can do ... for such the sole executant
> is muscle, whether in whispering a syllable or felling a forest.
>
> Charles Sherrington, in Sueng 2013

The Human Connectome Project aims to build a 'network map' that will shed light on the anatomical and functional connectivity within the brain. Sebastian Seung, in his book *Connectome: how the brain's wiring makes us who we are*,[11] explains that any kind of personal change is about changing your connectomes. Seung explains that, unlike our genome, which is fixed from the moment of conception, our connectomes change throughout life. There are many unknowns on the matter but it's largely believed that life experiences and genetics change our connectomes. Does this matter to our ultimate goals in IPC? Is there a way of influencing people's connectomes that we just haven't found yet? Will the outcome of the Human Connectome Project be helpful to us in the future? Seung describes the way muscles work, the axons, the synapses, contractions of fibres – muscles being the final destination of all neural pathways. This is of relevance in instilling habits. Neuroscientists explain that brain cells found where habits are formed and movement is controlled have receptors that work like computer processors to translate regular activities into habits.[12]

At a philosophical level, isn't this the ultimate goal of most of what we are doing in IPC – trying to facilitate, encourage, promote and make it as easy as possible for people to do certain things with their muscles – open their mouth and communicate in a certain way, hold a device in a certain way, reach out and press a plunger, put one hand on top of the other and move them together in a certain way and at the right time? A key aim of much of IPC is to translate learned behaviour into habitual behaviour, making it easy to perform certain tasks within a sea of complexity. Habits provide mental freedom and flexibility by enabling many activities to be on autopilot while the brain focuses on more urgent matters.[13] To date, much of this thinking is being used for tackling disease processes and addictions. However, in a field where habitual behaviours are wanted and sought after, there is much to learn from our colleagues in neuroscience. In the words of Tsien[13]:

> If you know cell circuits controlling a specific habit, it puts you in a better position to devise strategies to hit different points and selectively facilitate the formation of a good habit and maybe even reverse a bad one.

This may all seem rather random, but Seung[11] suggests that in the future it might even be possible to change connectomes such that we move away from traditional training to influence behaviours and thoughts, and move to new, more powerful approaches to enhance learning regimens. Our community would be foolish to ignore developments such as these that might aid how we maximise our influence in the pursuit of safer health and social care.

THE DARK ARTS: HYPNOTHERAPY AND NEUROLINGUISTIC PROGRAMMING

Hypnotherapy and NLP are often greatly misunderstood, their theoretical base the subject of question and until recently seen as separate to the mainstream of healthcare. For example, people confuse the clinical intervention of hypnotherapy with the entertaining (or not) endeavours of stage hypnotists. NLP is often criticised as being manipulative.

However, at a simplistic level, the clinical hypnotherapy part of the field of cognitive neuroscience can be described as the art of securing a person's attention and then effectively communicating ideas that enhance motivation and change perceptions.[14] In recent times its utility has grown in prominence as one method for addressing a range of clinical problems and unwanted habits. A number of high-profile individuals, from David Beckham to Tiger Woods, have openly talked of its use as a means of enhancing sports performance. What, therefore, can we learn from clinical hypnotherapy in our role as teachers, trainers and influencers?

Hypnosis classically refers to a change in baseline mental activity following an induction procedure[15] – more widely described as putting a person into a trance. The purpose of hypnotic induction is to *warm up* an individual to be more responsive to suggestion, the suggestions often relating to desired or unwanted behaviours. In relation to performance, a technique known as 'anchoring' can be used to instil a behaviour within a person's subconscious and associate it with a certain action so that, when conscious, the action will bring back the desired performance in an automatic way.

I am not suggesting that we use mass trance-inducing sessions as part of the routine training of health workers or, indeed, any aspect of conventional clinical hypnosis within IPC. What I am suggesting is that those of us interested in taking the next steps in terms of understanding human behaviour and habit formation and breaking, should be exposed to the art and science of hypnotherapy. I believe it has much to offer in how we influence colleagues, how we talk, how we teach and the words we use and how we say them.

NLP is equally fascinating in its potential to strengthen what we do and how we do it. Described as an emerging technology in healthcare, NLP is a relatively new approach to communication and personal development that has been increasingly used in education and teaching.[16] However, as with hypnotherapy, up until recently there has been little academic work in this area. Tosey *et al.*[16] describe NLP as an innovation and explain that it is concerned with the connections between a person's internal experience (neuro), their language (linguistic) and their patterns of behaviour (programming). In essence, NLP is a form of modelling that has meaningful implications for training. It offers a communication framework using techniques to understand and facilitate change in thinking and behaviour by proposing that a person's internal representations of the world show a bias for a particular sensory modality (visual, auditory, kinaesthetic, olfactory or gustatory).[17]

WHAT CAN WE DO WITH THIS?

The relevance and application of behavioural theories per se in IPC is context specific. Some of the alternative approaches described here require further development. However, the intention is to stimulate thinking beyond the conventional comfortable world that we exist in and consider how some of the techniques that are used in hypnotherapy and NLP might enhance part of what IPC does to influence behaviour.

Drawing on the Behaviour Change Wheel and elements of the World Health Organization's multimodal strategy, and considering the role that hypnotherapy and NLP might have in influencing behaviour, consider the following three questions:
1. How might we enhance education and training?
2. How might we stimulate action at the bedside, e.g. with reference to hand hygiene or insertion of an intravenous device?
3. How might we engage our colleagues in day-to-day conversation amidst the competing demands and general 'noise'?

In Table 11.1 I propose a number of suggestions, but you might have your own; neither is wrong.

TABLE 11.1 Some suggestions for applying neuroscience to infection prevention and control

Question	Suggestion
How might we enhance education and training?	• Using techniques of hypnotherapy to reinforce behaviours, e.g. use of language, repetition and tone of voice, to deliver short (50-second) effective educational sessions such as podcasts, short YouTube channel videos • Draw on the principles of hypnotherapeutic ego-strengthening techniques to motivate people to feel good about doing the right thing
How might we stimulate action at the bedside, e.g. with reference to hand hygiene or insertion of an intravenous device?	• Hypnotherapeutic installation of cues to persuade people to perform a set action in response to a specific stimulus: — e.g. every time you … see a patient as you enter the patient zone, you will immediately, without thinking, reach out and clean your hands — e.g. every time you go to perform a clean or aseptic task you will immediately … • The system as a cue to action, e.g. install cues so that every time a health worker sees a certain physical product a desired action is stimulated

(continued)

Question	Suggestion
How might we engage our colleagues in day-to-day conversation amidst the competing demands and general 'noise'?	• Training on NLP modalities or other effective communication approaches based on how the brain functions, to encourage the right language for impact, depending on the target audience

Each of the questions posed in Table 11.1 are concerned to varying degrees with affecting the capability, opportunity and motivation of the target audience as per Michie *et al.*'s[6] Behaviour Change Wheel. My suggestions are designed to stimulate thinking in those of you who are looking for new ideas to explore. At this stage these remain ideas, but based on my understanding and experience of clinical hypnotherapy and NLP I think these two disciplines have much to teach us in IPC. They are not the solution, but some of the insights they provide are at the very least fascinating and at best could be of practical use.

KEY REFLECTIONS

In concluding this chapter I present a number of points for your reflection.

- Do we have the right skills to develop policies, protocols, training materials and messages to affect behaviour of our multiple target audiences?
- Is it necessary to develop a field of science that covers neuro-IPC or behavioural IPC?
- If so, how far are we from appointing the first neuro- or behavioural infection preventionist?
- How could undergraduate and postgraduate training of all disciplines be improved to incorporate neurosciences and behavioural IPC?
- Are we clear which of the behaviours that we need to influence are open to modification?
- Do we design the workplace to take account of the brain and behaviour and its influence on habits?

I'm not sure what percentage of the nearly 3000 words that precede the one you're reading right now hold any sort of key to unlocking some of the answers that have as yet eluded us in the specialty of IPC. However, I suggest that some of the principles and techniques associated with, in particular, NLP and hypnotherapy may have a place in enhancing IPC. Relying on conventional methods and placing too much weight on training and policy writing without appreciating the complexity of behaviour change is folly. As one author reminds us, the brain really is wider than the sky[18] and what is certain is that conventional approaches have as yet failed to provide all of the answers. If you really want to penetrate even a handful of the 100 billion neurons that make up the brain of the next person you're trying to influence, pause for a moment to consider how much of the social sciences have formed the foundation of the advice you give, the policy you have written or the training package you've recently constructed.

REFERENCES

1. Edwards R, Charani E, Sevdalis N, *et al*. Optimisation of infection prevention and control in acute health care by use of behaviour change: a systematic review. *Lancet Infect Dis*. 2012; **12**(4): 318–29.
2. Elliott P. *Infection Control: a psychosocial approach to changing practice*. Oxford: Radcliffe; 2009.
3. World Health Organization (WHO). *WHO Guidelines on Hand Hygiene in Health Care*. Geneva: WHO; 2009.
4. Jenner EA, Watson PWB, Miller L, *et al*. Explaining hand hygiene practice: an extended application of the theory of planned behaviour. *Psychol Health Med*. 2002; **7**(3): 311–26
5. Curry V, Cole M. Applying social and behavioral theory as a template in containing and confining VRE. *Crit Care Nurs Q*. 2001 Aug; **24**(2): 13–19.
6. Michie S, van Stralen MM, West R. The Behaviour Change Wheel: a new method for characterising and designing behaviour change interventions. *Implement Sci*. 2011; **6**: 42.
7. Grist M. *Steer: mastering our behaviour through instinct, environment and reason*. London: RSA; 2010.
8. White C. Nudging, fishing, and improving the public's health. *BMJ*. 2011; **343**: d8046.
9. Kahneman D. *Thinking, Fast and Slow*. London: Penguin Books; 2012.
10. Storr J, Wigglesworth N, Kilpatrick C. *Integrating Human Factors with Infection Prevention and Control*. Thought Paper. London: The Health Foundation; 2013. Available at: www. health.org.uk/publication/integrating-human-factors-infection-prevention-and-control (accessed 25 June 2015).
11. Seung S. *Connectome: how the brain's wiring makes us who we are*. New York, NY: Houghton Mifflin Harcourt; 2013.
12. Wang LP, Li F, Wang D, *et al*. NMDA receptors in dopaminergic neurons are crucial for habit learning. *Neuron*. 2011; **72**(6): 1055–66.
13. Georgia Health Sciences University. *Habit Formation is Enabled by Gateway to Brain Cells*. ScienceDaily. 2012 Jan 13. Available at: www.sciencedaily.com/releases/2011/12/111221140448.htm (accessed 14 March 2015).
14. Crasilneck HB. *Handbook of Hypnotic Suggestions and Metaphors*. New York, NY: WW Norton; 1990.
15. Oakley DA, Halligan PW. Hypnotic suggestion and cognitive neuroscience. *Trends Cogn Sci*. 2009; **13**(6): 264–70.
16. Tosey P, Mathison J. *Neuro-Linguistic Programming: its potential for learning and teaching in formal education*. Paper presented at the European Conference on Educational Research,

University of Hamburg, 17–20 September 2003. Available at: www.leeds.ac.uk/educol/documents/00003319.htm (accessed 14 March 2015).

17. Sturt J, Ali S, Robertson W, *et al.* Neurolinguistic programming: a systematic review of the effects on health outcomes. *Br J Gen Pract.* 2012; **62**(604): e757–64.

18. Appleyard B. *The Brain is Wider than the Sky: why simple solutions don't work in a complex world.* London: Weidenfeld & Nicolson; 2012.

CHAPTER 12

Infection prevention and control education and training: research findings and an electronic learning experience for undergraduate students

....

Debra Teasdale and Paul Elliott

We would like to start by asking you to reflect on the following three questions.

1. To what degree do you feel the education and training you have received, if any, into infection prevention and control (IP&C) has influenced the way you adhere to standard precautions within your professional practice?

2. To what degree do you feel the education and training you have received, if any, into IP&C has served to enhance your understanding of the importance of adopting standard precautions?

3. On a broader perspective, to what extent do you feel IP&C education has contributed to reductions in cross-infection?

Historically, the importance of appropriate IP&C education and training as a means of facilitating safe practice has been well documented.[1-5] Further, it has also been documented that IP&C education and training has been deficient in its frequency and methods of delivery as a means of producing identifiable reductions in cross-infection,[6,7] and that many of those involved in the provision of health and social care have been significantly negligent in their undertaking of safe IP&C. A disturbing case in point within the British National Health Service being highlighted within the 'Francis Report',[8] where it appears that IP&C violations were occurring over an extended period of time. In some ways it would seem that we have progressed little over the past 200 years, as is borne out by the immortal words of Florence Nightingale:

> I take leave to give the facts, we wait for the rates of mortality to go up before we interfere and when enough have died we enter the results of our masterly activity neatly in tables, but we do not analyse and tabulate the saddened lives of those who remain ...[9]

Further, Miss Nightingale believed in the importance of education as something that would serve to promote appropriate standards of hygiene.[9] Yet, some 200 years on it would seem that education and training around IP&C and the subsequent undertaking of, for example, standard precautions, is paid little more than lip service where some health and social care professionals are concerned!* With this in mind, two examples from personal experience are given below.

Experience 1

While attending a psychology conference several years ago I had a conversation with a psychologist who pronounced that they did not need to worry about IP&C because they did not touch their clients and that they saw no need for psychologists to learn about IP&C, as it bore no relevance to their role.

Experience 2

Some years ago as a part of my lecturing role I had a conversation with an undergraduate student regarding IP&C. Part of this conversation involved the importance of undertaking appropriate IP&C practice. As a part of this conversation, the student stated that, as they were not a nurse, they did not need to worry about IP&C. They reasoned that this was because, first, they did not touch their clients; second, their tutor had told them that infection could

---

* Where reference is made to health and social care it is intended to include such professions as psychology, sociology, environmental and occupational health, and health promotion.

only be spread by touching someone; and third, there was little point in them bothering with any IP&C education and training, as it would not be needed.

Such perspectives not only demonstrate limited thinking but are inherently dangerous where the potential for cross infection is concerned.

With regard to both of these experiences, although it is acknowledged that they are subjective in nature, it would seem reasonable to identify a complete lack of understanding regarding the nature of cross-infection on the part of all three individuals (the psychologist, the student and the tutor). Further, regarding the apparent attitudes and beliefs of these individuals, the word irresponsible would seem to constitute somewhat of an understatement, bearing in mind that they would be placing not only themselves and those they allegedly care about at risk but also their colleagues and the general population at large. Clearly, both the undergraduate student and the psychologist appeared to perceive IP&C education and training as being of little value.

In 1989, Elliott[10] identified, from a participant-administered survey relating to undergraduate nursing, medicine and the allied health professions, that the emphasis placed upon hand hygiene education was inconsistent and lacked any uniformity, although some respondents did acknowledge that hand hygiene was covered at some point during their programme of professional education. In 1994, Gould and Chamberlain[11] identified the importance of clinically based education around IP&C and that such education should be a collaborative venture between academia and practice. In 1996, Elliott[12] undertook a further participant-administered survey, this time within a Welsh district general hospital where staff were asked from whom their hand hygiene was first learned following the commencement of their undergraduate programme of professional education. Of the 350 individuals surveyed, 63 (or 18%) identified they had received no education at all. In other words, they made it up as they went along! Although 63 out of 350 may seem a small number, consideration must be given to the potential that these 63 individuals may have contributed to cross-infection rates, and that these individuals received no education at all might infer that those responsible for the provision of education failed in their duty of care by default. Further, as a part of the same research, 20 centres of nurse education were contacted with regard to their policy on hand hygiene education, to which there were three overriding responses (see List 12.1).

LIST 12.1 Overriding responses[12]

- Education was undertaken through researching recent literature with no lecturer or IP&C specialist input.
- Education was undertaken through constant reminders but these were infrequent and not evidence based.
- Hand hygiene education was allocated between 3 and 21 hours over the period of their undergraduate programme of professional education.

Clearly none of these overriding responses could be perceived as being either valid or reliable where reducing the risk of cross-infection was concerned. Further, the findings of this survey identified that, for the most part, clinical practitioners were excluded from the IP&C educational process.

In 2000, Sherertz et al.[13] identified that instruction into IP&C varied widely. They further indicated that the principle of 'see one, do one, teach one' can lead to inconsistencies in the ways procedures are undertaken. Further, Hallett[14] has indicated that education may create a sense of ambivalence and uncertainty with regard to infection control, and particularly so where wound care is concerned. Clearly, the negating of such ambivalence and uncertainty is vital if IP&C is to be undertaken appropriately, which must in part have implications for the methods used to facilitate such learning. For example, the 'see one, do one, teach one' method could well have inconsistencies between what is perceived to be appropriate by those adopting such a method of learning. Certainly, Rosenthal et al.[15] showed that education and clinical training could result in improved levels of compliance with regard to IP&C.

In light of the findings mentioned and the development of a new curriculum within the Faculty of Health and Wellbeing at Canterbury Christ Church University, an electronic participant-administered survey where 20 centres of nurse education within the United Kingdom were contacted to ascertain the emphasis they placed upon the education and clinical training of IP&C, and who, if anyone, undertook such with regard to their undergraduate students.[16] From this survey a number of principle findings were established (see List 12.2).

From that outlined within List 12.2 it was deduced at the time (2008) that the knowledge base of student nurses – during their programme of professional education, upon initial qualification and initial entry to the Nursing and Midwifery Council's Professional Register – in relation to IP&C might well be somewhat concerning. Further, some of the findings identified within List 12.2 would seem to reflect those found by Elliott in 1996[12] some 11 years earlier.

LIST 12.2 United Kingdom centres of nurse education[16]

- Overall the provision of IP&C education was significantly lacking.
- The approach to IP&C was:
  - no education at all
  - once at the beginning of year 1
  - left solely to the mentors and staff within clinical placements
  - student-led, self-directed study
  - through a single lecture with no skills laboratory practical time
  - IP&C knowledge and skills not assessed
  - IP&C clinical specialists generally excluded from any type of education that did occur.

LIST 12.3 ICPLE overview[17]

Year 1

The aim of this was to provide students with a grounding in the principles of infection prevention and control.

Year 2

The aim of this was to introduce students to the psychological and social aspects of infection prevention and control.

Year 3

During this year students undertook a project of their own choosing and were required to present the project to their personal tutor at the end of year 3.

Following these findings (List 12.2) and the recognition at Canterbury Christ Church University that there needed to be put in place some form of IP&C learning experience, the findings were presented to the Faculty of Health and Wellbeing, and those with responsibility for IP&C within the School of Nursing developed as a part of a new curriculum for 2009 such a learning experience. Subsequently, in 2009 an electronic Infection Control and Prevention Learning Experience (ICPLE)[17] went live for pre-registration health and social care students (*see* List 12.3).

In 2012, after the ICPLE element of students' professional education had run for 3 years, Teasdale and Elliott undertook a pilot study to investigate the degree to which undergraduate students complied with the five-stage hand hygiene process,[18] which is a vital element of the ICPLE. The essential elements of this study are outlined in Tables 12.1, 12.2, 12.3 and 12.4.

TABLE 12.1 Pathway of professional education

Pathway	Number of students
Adult Nursing	56
Child Nursing	17
Speech and Language Therapy	14
Midwifery	11
Operating Department Practitioner	2
Occupational Therapy	1
Radiography	1
Total	**102**

TABLE 12.2 Year of professional education

Year	Number of students
Year 1	75
Year 2	26
Year 3	1
Total	**102**

TABLE 12.3 Ethnic origin as indicated by the student

Ethnic origin	Number of students
British	79
African	5
Irish	4
European	3
Caribbean	2
Caucasian	2
Indian	2
Danish	1

(continued)

Ethnic origin	Number of students
Filipino	1
Nepalese	1
South American	1
No response	1
Total	**102**

TABLE 12.4 Age and gender

Age	Female	Male	Total
17–20	33		33
21–25	26	3	29
26–30	11	2	13
31–35	11		11
36–40	8		8
41–45	3		3
46–50	4		4
50+	1		1
Totals	**97**	**5**	**102**

ETHICAL APPROVAL

Ethical approval was sought and obtained through the Faculty of Health and Wellbeing Ethics Committee at Canterbury Christ Church University, and students were recruited on a volunteer basis through posters and electronic media. Having volunteered, the aim of the pilot study was fully explained and students then had the option to withdraw if they wished; none did so. For the 102 students who took part in the study, they were each given a £3 voucher that they could spend within any of the university's cafeterias.

METHODOLOGY

The study was undertaken within one of two skills laboratories, depending upon where students were based. Each student was simply instructed by an observer to undertake hand hygiene as he or she would normally do while working within a clinical practice setting. Following that, no further communication took place between the observer and the student. While the student undertook his or her hand hygiene, the observer completed a prepared record sheet (see List 12.3).

LIST 12.3 Hand hygiene process adherence checklist

Observer instructions

1. You should observe the participant undertaking hand hygiene and record the participant's adherence to the hand hygiene process as identified in the checklist.
2. As the observer you are not looking to assess the participant's hand hygiene technique, only his or her adherence to the stages of the hand hygiene process identified.
3. Place a number from 1 to 5 in the 'stage' boxes to indicate the sequence in which the participant adopted the stages of the hand hygiene process.
4. Adherence to the process is only determined if the participant follows the five stages of the process in the correct sequence.
5. If the participant deviates in any way from the correct sequence, then that should be classed as non-adherence.
6. At the bottom of the sheet circle either Adherence or Non-Adherence, in accordance with the participant's undertaking of the hand hygiene process.

Prelim stage: removes watch, rings and rolls sleeves up?

Watch:	Yes/No
Rings:	Yes/No
Sleeves rolled up:	Yes/No

Stage 1: wetting of the hands and wrists with running water ☐

Stage 2: application of the cleansing solution ☐

Stage 3: washing of the hand and wrists (minimum time of 15 seconds) ☐

Stage 4: thorough rinsing of the areas washed under running water (including under rings if not removed) ☐

Stage 5: thorough drying of the areas washed with disposable hand towels ☐

Additional information

Note the number of disposable towels used to dry the hands ☐

Shake hands with participant to determine if hands are dry or still wet (D = dry; W = wet) ☐

Overall result

ADHERENCE _____   NON-ADHERENCE _____

RESULTS

Adherence to the five-stage hand hygiene process

Of the 102 students who took part in the study, 81 adhered fully to the five-stage hand hygiene process in the correct sequence, while 21 students deviated from the correct sequence.

Effective drying of the hands

Of the 102 students who took part, 20 were deemed to have dried their hands appropriately, while 82 were deemed to have failed to do so. The method of drying was disposable paper towels. The effectiveness of hand drying was ascertained by the observer shaking the hands of the students afterwards. If the student's hands were anything other than felt to be completely dry, this was recorded as a failure to dry the hands thoroughly.

Removal of wristwatches prior to commencing hand hygiene

Of the 102 students who took part and wore wristwatches, 15 removed them prior to commencing hand hygiene, while 13 students failed to remove their wristwatches prior to commencing hand hygiene. The remaining 74 students were not wearing wristwatches and this is indicated by the word 'None' within the wristwatch column in Table 12.5.

Removal of rings prior to commencing hand hygiene

Of the 102 students who took part and were wearing rings, 14 removed them prior to commencing hand hygiene, while 25 students failed to remove their rings prior to commencing hand hygiene. the remaining 63 students were not wearing rings and this is indicated by the use of the word 'None' within the rings column in Table 12.5.

Sleeves above the elbow

Of the 102 students who took part and had sleeves below the elbow, 67 rolled the up above the elbow prior to commencing hand hygiene, while 17 students undertook hand hygiene with their sleeves below the elbow. The remaining 18 students were already wearing clothing that had sleeves above the elbow and this is indicated by the use of the word 'None' within the sleeves column in Table 12.5.

TABLE 12.5 Complete data set

No.	Age	Gender	Location	Pathway	Education	Ethnic origin	Watch	Rings	Sleeves	S1	S2	S3	S4	S5	No. of towels	Hands	Adherence to the hand hygiene process
1	26–30	F	Canterbury	Midwifery	Year2	Caucasian	None	No	Yes	1	2	3	4	5	2	Wet	Yes
2	36–40	F	Canterbury	Midwifery	Year2	British	None	None	Yes	2	1	3	4	5	2	Wet	No
3	26–30	F	Canterbury	Midwifery	Year2	European	None	No	Yes	1	2	3	4	5	2	Dry	Yes
4	21–25	F	Canterbury	Midwifery	Year2	British	None	None	Yes	1	2	3	4	5	3	Wet	Yes
5	21–25	F	Canterbury	Midwifery	Year2	British	Yes	Yes	Yes	1	2	3	4	5	2	Wet	Yes
6	17–20	F	Canterbury	Midwifery	Year2	British	None	None	Yes	1	2	3	4	5	2	Wet	Yes
7	17–20	F	Canterbury	Midwifery	Year2	British	None	Yes	No	1	2	3	4	5	4	Wet	Yes
8	17–20	F	Canterbury	Midwifery	Year2	British	No	No	Yes	1	2	3	4	5	3	Dry	Yes
9	21–25	F	Canterbury	Midwifery	Year2	British	No	None	Yes	1	2	3	4	5	2	Wet	Yes
10	17–20	F	Canterbury	Midwifery	Year2	British	None	None	None	1	2	3	4	5	3	Dry	Yes
11	21–25	F	Canterbury	Midwifery	Year2	British	None	None	Yes	1	2	3	4	5	3	Wet	Yes
12	17–20	F	Canterbury	Child Nursing	Year1	British	None	None	None	0	1	2	3	4	4	Wet	No
13	17–20	F	Canterbury	Child Nursing	Year1	British	None	None	None	1	2	3	4	5	4	Wet	Yes
14	17–20	F	Canterbury	Child Nursing	Year1	British	None	None	None	1	2	3	4	5	5	Dry	Yes
15	17–20	F	Canterbury	Child Nursing	Year1	Not Given	None	None	None	1	2	3	4	5	2	Wet	Yes
16	17–20	F	Canterbury	Child Nursing	Year1	British	None	None	None	1	2	3	0	5	2	Wet	No
17	21–25	F	Canterbury	Child Nursing	Year1	British	None	None	None	1	2	3	4	5	1	Wet	Yes
18	17–20	F	Canterbury	Child Nursing	Year1	British	None	None	None	1	2	3	4	5	3	Dry	Yes
19	17–20	F	Canterbury	Child Nursing	Year1	British	None	None	None	1	2	3	4	5	3	Wet	Yes
20	17–20	F	Canterbury	Child Nursing	Year1	British	None	None	None	1	2	3	4	5	2	Wet	Yes

No.	Age	Gender	Location	Pathway	Education	Ethnic origin	Watch	Rings	Sleeves	S1	S2	S3	S4	S5	No. of towels	Hands	Adherence to the hand hygiene process
21	21–25	F	Canterbury	Child Nursing	Year1	British	None	None	None	1	2	3	4	5	3	Wet	Yes
22	21–25	F	Canterbury	Child Nursing	Year1	British	None	None	None	1	2	3	4	5	3	Dry	Yes
23	26–30	F	Canterbury	Child Nursing	Year1	British	None	None	None	2	1	3	4	5	2	Wet	No
24	17–20	F	Canterbury	Child Nursing	Year1	British	None	None	None	1	2	3	0	5	2	Wet	No
25	17–20	F	Canterbury	Child Nursing	Year1	British	None	None	None	0	1	2	3	4	2	Wet	No
26	21–25	F	Canterbury	Child Nursing	Year1	African	None	None	None	1	2	3	4	5	3	Wet	Yes
27	17–20	F	Canterbury	Adult Nursing	Year2	British	None	None	None	1	2	3	4	5	4	Wet	Yes
28	17–20	F	Canterbury	Adult Nursing	Year2	British	Yes	Yes	Yes	1	2	3	4	5	3	Wet	Yes
29	17–20	F	Canterbury	Adult Nursing	Year2	British	Yes	Yes	None	1	2	3	4	5	3	Wet	Yes
30	17–20	F	Canterbury	Adult Nursing	Year2	British	None	None	Yes	1	2	3	4	5	4	Dry	Yes
31	26–30	F	Canterbury	Radiography	Year2	British	Yes	Yes	Yes	1	2	3	4	5	3	Wet	Yes
32	46–50	F	Canterbury	Occupational Therapy	Year2	British	None	No	Yes	1	2	3	4	5	3	Wet	Yes
33	50+	F	Canterbury	Adult Nursing	Year2	Caucasian	Yes	Yes	Yes	1	2	3	4	5	5	Wet	Yes
34	31–35	F	Canterbury	Adult Nursing	Year1	European	Yes	Yes	Yes	1	2	3	4	5	2	0	Yes
35	21–25	F	Chatham	Adult Nursing	Year1	British	None	No	Yes	2	1	3	4	5	5	Wet	No
36	21–25	F	Canterbury	Adult Nursing	Year1	British	No	No	Yes	1	2	3	4	5	2	Wet	Yes
37	36–40	F	Chatham	Adult Nursing	Year1	Danish	Yes	None	Yes	1	2	3	4	5	2	Wet	Yes
38	36–40	F	Chatham	Adult Nursing	Year1	British	None	None	Yes	1	2	3	4	5	4	Wet	Yes
39	46–50	F	Chatham	Adult Nursing	Year1	British	Yes	No	No	1	2	3	4	5	5	Wet	Yes
40	26–30	M	Chatham	Adult Nursing	Year1	British	None	None	Yes	1	2	3	4	5	5	0	Yes
41	31–35	F	Chatham	Adult Nursing	Year1	British	None	None	Yes	1	2	3	4	5	4	Wet	Yes

No.	Age	Gender	Location	Pathway	Education	Ethnic origin	Watch	Rings	Sleeves	S1	S2	S3	S4	S5	No. of towels	Hands	Adherence to the hand hygiene process
42	41–45	F	Chatham	Adult Nursing	Year1	British	No	No	Yes	1	2	3	4	5	2	Wet	Yes
43	46–50	F	Canterbury	Adult Nursing	Year1	British	No	No	No	1	2	3	4	5	5	Wet	Yes
44	21–25	F	Canterbury	Adult Nursing	Year1	British	None	None	Yes	1	2	3	4	5	1	Wet	Yes
45	17–20	F	Canterbury	Adult Nursing	Year1	African	None	None	Yes	1	2	3	4	5	3	Wet	Yes
46	26–30	M	Canterbury	Adult Nursing	Year1	Indian	Yes	No	Yes	0	1	2	4	5	2	Wet	No
47	36–40	F	Canterbury	Adult Nursing	Year1	British	None	None	Yes	1	2	3	4	5	4	Wet	Yes
48	21–25	F	Canterbury	Adult Nursing	Year1	British	None	Yes	Yes	1	2	3	4	5	2	Wet	Yes
49	21–25	F	Canterbury	Adult Nursing	Year1	Nepalese	None	None	Yes	1	2	3	4	5	2	Wet	Yes
50	21–25	F	Canterbury	Adult Nursing	Year1	British	None	No	Yes	1	2	3	4	5	3	Wet	Yes
51	17–20	F	Canterbury	Adult Nursing	Year1	British	Yes	Yes	Yes	1	2	3	4	5	2	Wet	Yes
52	17–20	F	Canterbury	Adult Nursing	Year1	British	None	None	No	1	2	3	4	5	3	Wet	Yes
53	26–30	F	Canterbury	Adult Nursing	Year1	British	None	None	Yes	1	2	3	4	5	2	Wet	Yes
54	21–25	F	Canterbury	Adult Nursing	Year1	British	None	No	Yes	1	2	3	4	5	2	Wet	Yes
55	21–25	M	Canterbury	Adult Nursing	Year1	British	Yes	None	Yes	1	2	3	4	5	4	Dry	Yes
56	21–25	M	Canterbury	Adult Nursing	Year1	British	None	None	Yes	1	2	3	4	5	3	Wet	Yes
57	17–20	F	Canterbury	Adult Nursing	Year1	British	No	No	No	0	1	2	3	4	3	Wet	No
58	26–30	F	Canterbury	Adult Nursing	Year1	South American	None	No	Yes	1	2	3	4	5	2	Wet	Yes
59	26–30	F	Canterbury	Adult Nursing	Year1	Filipino	None	None	Yes	1	2	3	4	5	2	Dry	Yes
60	41–45	F	Canterbury	Adult Nursing	Year1	Caribbean	None	No	No	1	2	3	4	5	3	Dry	Yes
61	21–25	F	Canterbury	Adult Nursing	Year1	British	None	None	No	0	1	2	3	4	2	Wet	No
62	17–20	F	Canterbury	Adult Nursing	Year1	British	None	None	Yes	1	2	3	4	5	3	Wet	Yes

No.	Age	Gender	Location	Pathway	Education	Ethnic origin	Watch	Rings	Sleeves	S1	S2	S3	S4	S5	No. of towels	Hands	Adherence to the hand hygiene process
63	17–20	F	Canterbury	Adult Nursing	Year1	British	None	None	Yes	1	2	3	4	5	2	Wet	Yes
64	17–20	F	Canterbury	Adult Nursing	Year1	Irish	None	No	Yes	1	2	3	4	5	4	Wet	Yes
65	21–25	M	Canterbury	Adult Nursing	Year1	British	None	None	Yes	1	2	3	4	5	3	Wet	Yes
66	36–40	F	Canterbury	Adult Nursing	Year1	British	None	No	Yes	1	2	3	4	5	3	Dry	Yes
67	36–40	F	Canterbury	Adult Nursing	Year1	British	None	No	Yes	1	2	3	4	5	4	Dry	Yes
68	17–20	F	Canterbury	Adult Nursing	Year1	British	None	None	Yes	1	2	3	4	5	3	Wet	Yes
69	21–25	F	Canterbury	Adult Nursing	Year1	African	None	None	No	1	2	3	4	5	2	Wet	Yes
70	17–20	F	Canterbury	Adult Nursing	Year1	African	None	None	Yes	1	2	3	4	5	4	Dry	Yes
71	21–25	F	Canterbury	Adult Nursing	Year1	British	None	None	Yes	1	2	3	4	5	3	Wet	Yes
72	17–20	F	Canterbury	Adult Nursing	Year1	Irish	None	None	Yes	1	2	3	4	5	3	Wet	Yes
73	17–20	F	Canterbury	Adult Nursing	Year1	Irish	None	None	No	1	2	3	4	5	2	Dry	Yes
74	17–20	F	Canterbury	Adult Nursing	Year1	British	None	None	Yes	1	2	3	4	5	3	Wet	Yes
75	26–30	F	Canterbury	Adult Nursing	Year1	British	None	None	Yes	1	2	3	4	5	2	Wet	Yes
76	17–20	F	Canterbury	Adult Nursing	Year1	British	None	None	Yes	1	2	3	4	5	3	Wet	Yes
77	17–20	F	Canterbury	Adult Nursing	Year1	British	None	Yes	Yes	1	2	3	4	5	3	Wet	Yes
78	31–35	F	Canterbury	Adult Nursing	Year1	British	Yes	Yes	Yes	1	2	3	4	5	2	Dry	Yes
79	21–25	F	Canterbury	Adult Nursing	Year3	Irish	None	None	Yes	0	1	2	3	4	4	Wet	No
80	36–40	F	Chatham	Adult Nursing	Year2	British	None	No	No	1	2	3	4	5	2	Wet	Yes
81	31–35	F	Chatham	Speech and Language Therapy	Year1	British	No	None	No	1	2	3	4	5	2	Dry	Yes
82	31–35	F	Chatham	Speech and Language Therapy	Year1	Indian	None	None	No	0	1	2	3	4	3	Wet	No

No.	Age	Gender	Location	Pathway	Education	Ethnic origin	Watch	Rings	Sleeves	S1	S2	S3	S4	S5	No. of towels	Hands	Adherence to the hand hygiene process
83	21–25	F	Chatham	Speech and Language Therapy	Year1	British	None	No	Yes	0	1	2	3	4	2	Wet	No
84	41–45	F	Chatham	Speech and Language Therapy	Year1	British	No	No	No	1	2	3	4	5	3	Dry	Yes
85	21–25	F	Chatham	Speech and Language Therapy	Year1	British	None	None	Yes	0	1	2	3	4	4	Wet	No
86	26–30	F	Chatham	Speech and Language Therapy	Year1	British	Yes	No	Yes	1	2	3	4	5	2	Wet	Yes
87	46–50	F	Chatham	Speech and Language Therapy	Year1	British	None	None	Yes	0	1	2	3	4	3	Wet	No
88	21–25	F	Chatham	Speech and Language Therapy	Year1	African	Yes	None	Yes	1	2	3	4	5	2	Wet	Yes
89	21–25	F	Chatham	Speech and Language Therapy	Year1	British	No	No	Yes	1	2	3	4	5	2	Wet	Yes
90	26–30	F	Chatham	Speech and Language Therapy	Year1	British	None	None	Yes	1	2	3	4	5	2	Dry	Yes
91	21–25	F	Chatham	Speech and Language Therapy	Year1	Caribbean	No	None	No	0	1	2	3	4	2	Wet	No

No.	Age	Gender	Location	Pathway	Education	Ethnic origin	Watch	Rings	Sleeves	S1	S2	S3	S4	S5	No. of towels	Hands	Adherence to the hand hygiene process
92	21–25	F	Chatham	Speech and Language Therapy	Year1	British	No	None	No	0	1	2	3	4	2	Wet	No
93	31–35	F	Chatham	Speech and Language Therapy	Year1	British	No	Yes	No	0	1	2	3	4	3	Wet	No
94	26–30	F	Chatham	Operating Department Practitioner	Year2	British	Yes	Yes	Yes	1	2	3	4	5	2	Wet	Yes
95	31–35	F	Chatham	Speech and Language Therapy	Year1	British	No	No	Yes	1	2	3	4	5	4	Wet	Yes
96	31–35	F	Chatham	Operating Department Practitioner	Year2	European	None	None	Yes	1	2	3	4	5	2	Dry	Yes
97	17–20	F	Chatham	Adult Nursing	Year2	British	None	None	Yes	1	2	3	4	5	6	Wet	Yes
98	31–35	F	Chatham	Adult Nursing	Year1	British	None	No	Yes	0	1	2	3	4	3	Dry	No
99	31–35	F	Chatham	Child Nursing	Year2	British	None	Yes	Yes	1	2	3	4	5	2	Wet	Yes
100	21–25	F	Chatham	Child Nursing	Year2	British	None	None	No	0	1	2	3	4	2	Wet	No
101	36–40	F	Chatham	Adult Nursing	Year2	British	None	None	Yes	0	1	2	3	4	3	Wet	No

Notes: S1, S2, S3, S4, S5 = stages of the hand hygiene process. (Stage 1 = wetting of the hands and wrists under running water; Stage 2 = applying of the cleansing solution to the hands; Stage 3 = washing of the hands and wrists for a minimum of 15 seconds; Stage 4 = rinsing of the hands and wrists with running water; Stage 5 = drying of the hands with disposable paper towels.) Within S1–S5, if a '0' is presented, this means that this activity was not undertaken at all. The presentation of numbers within S1–S5 indicates the sequence in which the hand hygiene activities were undertaken. Within the gender column, F = female student, M = male student. Within the education column, the year = stage of professional education.

LIMITATIONS OF THE STUDY

- It is acknowledged that the Hawthorne effect could have been an influencing factor regarding the students' hand hygiene behaviour, and particularly so as the two observers were lecturing staff.
- It is also acknowledged that the method used to assess drying of the students' hands was a subjective measure and open to personal interpretation of the two observers.
- The sample size was very small and as such could not be taken as representative of the undergraduate health and social care student population.
- It is acknowledged that the £3 voucher could have had an influencing effect upon those students who agreed to take part.

FOLLOW-UP

Following completion of this study it was recognised that although the hand hygiene-related practice of some students was acceptable, there were others who clearly did not adhere to a safe approach to undertaking the hand hygiene process as set out in Table 12.5. Therefore, in view of these deviations from appropriate practice and following discussion among those with a remit for IP&C within the School of Nursing, the following points in List 12.4 were developed as a means of further facilitating appropriate adherence.

LIST 12.4 Actions to facilitate enhanced IP&C knowledge, skills and attitudes

1. A full review of the existing ICPLE should be undertaken and the content modified and updated where appropriate.
2. The ICPLE should become a part of the working agenda of the Undergraduate Programme Management Committee and the Curriculum Implementation Group, and regular reports should be presented to both of these groups by the Director of Clinical Practice within the School of Nursing.
3. The ICPLE should become an integral part of designated clinical practice-related modules within years 1, 2 and 3 of the students' programme of professional education.
4. The ICPLE should become part of the summative assessment of these designated clinical practice modules.
5. During the initial part of the students' professional education, prior to starting their clinical practice experience, and in conjunction with the module (*see*

---

point 3), students will spend time in the university's skills laboratories, where they will be given the opportunity to put theory into practice within a simulation setting under the supervision of both lecturing and clinical practitioners.

6. An IP&C committee should be established, with the membership consisting of both academics and clinical practitioners.

LIST 12.5 Examples from the revised ICPLE content[17]

Year 1

- Defining IP&C
- Standard precautions including hand hygiene
- Risks and sources of cross-infection
- Types of infectious agents
- The nature of cross-infection
- Sources of cross-infection and modes of transmission
- The chain of infection versus a unified approach to cross-infection[18]
- The impact of communication upon IP&C
- Legal issues in IP&C

Year 2

- Defining the psychosocial nature of IP&C
- Biomedical and biopsychosocial[19] approaches to IP&C
- Psychosocial theories that underpin IP&C
- The impact of attitudes, beliefs and stereotyping upon IP&C practice
- Factors that affect safe IP&C practice
- Cognition and IP&C behaviour

Year 3

During this final year of the programme of professional education, students should carry out an IP&C project.

- Project Part 1: Outline the project you intend to undertake.
- Project Part 2: Outline the methods you used to undertake your project.
- Project Part 3: Present the results of your project and how you intend to use your findings to enhance IP&C.

CONCLUSION

For all 3 years of the ICPLE[17] there is an integration of theory and practice, and students are expected to involve both relevant lecturers at the University and their mentor(s) in clinical practice. Students are also expected to reference elements of the work they produce, which must then be presented to their personal tutors at the end of each academic year. In addition, students' ICPLE work will be summatively assessed both in both theory and practice within a specifically designed and established Skills Laboratory Ward area at the University. In the years that the ICPLE programme has been running as an integral part of students' professional education, all undergraduate students have had access to such, but only Adult Nursing has embraced it as a means of facilitating their knowledge, skills and attitudes toward IP&C.

In concluding this chapter, it has been our intention to undertake a brief review of IP&C education and to reflect upon the nature of the IP&C education and clinical training that undergraduate health and social care students have available to them at Canterbury Christ Church University. In doing this, an evidence-based approach has been adopted that involves practitioners from both academia and clinical practice, with the aim of providing undergraduate health and social care students with both a good working knowledge of IP&C at the end of their 3-year programme and the opportunity to present or publish their year 3 project findings. Currently, based upon available information for 2014, Canterbury Christ Church University is a leading centre of professional education with regard to offering their health and social care students with such an extensive learning opportunity around IP&C.

REFERENCES

1. Gallagher R. Infection control: public health, clinical effectiveness and education. *Br J Nurs.* 1999; **8**(18): 1212–14.
2. Eggimann P, Pittet D. Overview of catheter-related infections with special emphasis on prevention based on educational programs. *Clin Microbiol Infect.* 2002; **8**(5): 295–309.
3. Voss A, Allerberger F, Bouza E, *et al.* The training curriculum in hospital infection control. *Clin Microbiol Infect.* 2005; **11**(Suppl. 1): 33–5.
4. Ward D. The role of education in the prevention and control of infection: a review of the literature. *Nurse Educ Today.* 2011; 31: 9–17.
5. Pfaff S. Education: past, present and future. *Am J Infect Control.* 1982; **10**(4): 133–7.
6. Cohen H, Kitai E, Levy I, *et al.* Handwashing patterns in two dermatology clinics. *Dermatology.* 2002; **205**(4): 258–361.
7. Wu C, Gardner G, Chang A. Nursing students' knowledge and practice of infection control precautions: an educational intervention. *J Adv Nurs.* 2009; **65**(10): 2142–9.

8. Francis R. The Mid Staffordshire NHS Foundation Trust Public Inquiry. London: The Mid Staffordshire NHS Foundation Trust; 2013. Available at: www.midstaffspublicinquiry.com/report (accessed 9 January 2015).

9. Ridgely Seymer L, editor. *Selected Writings of Florence Nightingale*. New York, NY: Macmillan; 1954.

10. Elliott P. To wash or not to wash? *Nurs Standard.* 1989; **36**(3): 21–3.

11. Gould G, Chamberlain A. Infection control as a topic for ward-based nursing education. *J Adv Nursing.* 1994; **20**: 275–82.

12. Elliott P. Handwashing practice in nurse education. *Prof Nurse.* 1996; **11**(6): 357–60.

13. Sherertz R, Ely E, Westbrook D, *et al.* Education of physicians-in-training can decrease the risk for vascular catheter infection. *Ann Intern Med.* 2000; **132**: 641–8.

14. Hallett C. Infection control in wound care: a study of fatalism in community nursing. *J Clin Nurs.* 2000; **9**: 103–9.

15. Rosenthal V. Effect of education and performance feedback on rates of catheter-associated urinary tract infection in intensive care units in Argentina. *Infect Control Hosp Epidemiol.* 2004; **25**(1): 47–50.

16. Clark S, Elliott P. *Report and Recommendations on Infection Prevention and Control Knowledge and Skills Acquisition for a New Pre-registration Curriculum in 2009.* Kent: Faculty of Health and Wellbeing, Canterbury Christ Church University; 2008.

17. Elliott P; Faculty of Health and Wellbeing, Canterbury Christ Church University. *Infection Prevention and Control Learning Experience (ICPLE).* Kent: Faculty of Health and Wellbeing, Canterbury Christ Church University; 2014.

18. Elliott P, editor. *Infection Control: a psychosocial approach to changing practice.* Abingdon: Radcliffe; 2009. pp. 12–14, 69.

19. Ogden J. *Health Psychology: a textbook.* 5th ed. Maidenhead: McGraw-Hill/Open University Press; 2012. pp. 4–7.

CHAPTER 13

Increasing the value and influence of infection prevention and control specialists

. . . .

Annette Jeanes

INTRODUCTION

Infection control is perceived by some as a one-issue service or specialty. Many infection control practitioners are narrowly focused on their specialty – in particular, compliance with controls and responses to infection-related events. In this chapter, the potential for infection prevention and control specialists (IPCSs) to have a wider influence on standards in healthcare services and add value to their role will be explored.

This chapter is designed to provide a starting point to improving the influence and value of IPCSs. The following issues will be covered:

- barriers and opportunities
- the potential for synergy in working practice
- upholding standards or 'being there'
- increasing influence
- super specialists
- self-efficacy
- value of influence.

BARRIERS AND OPPORTUNITIES

Translating the potential to influence change into the delivery of improved outcomes is a recognised challenge.[1] One of the barriers is that some ICPSs are comfortable working in a specialty with clear boundaries and so avoid encroachment into other areas such as risk and quality. Emersion in the specialism can act as a justification for not commenting, interacting, reflecting, making judgements or suggesting change in other areas of practice. ICPS may believe they have insufficient expertise or experience to influence areas of practice outside their specialty. Equally because they limit their scope this becomes a self-fulfilling prophesy.

It could also be argued that there is quite enough in this specialty to keep specialists occupied. Indeed, the number of IPCSs has grown considerably in the last decade, in response to the increased requirements and expectations of healthcare organisations.[2] The imposition of numerous guidelines, standards, audit and targets consume considerable time and effort, not just to produce them but also to translate them into changes in practice.[3]

As a specialty that frequently covers whole organisations, including many non-clinical areas that support care delivery, IPCSs are in a unique position. Few other healthcare workers are able to legitimately access such a broad range of services and staff with relative ease. Services can range from general practitioner surgeries, dentists, operating theatres, mortuary, hospital wards, laboratories, engineering plant, waste disposal collection bays, kitchens, sterile services department, outpatients and radiology. There is also a range of opportunities to interact with staff from numerous areas or organisations on visits, consultations and meetings – such as major incident planning groups, product selection groups, building planning groups, and risk and quality meetings.

The ability of infection prevention and control staff to respond to numerous and various situations may result in questions poised to infection prevention and control practitioners or observations made that are not directly related to infection prevention and control. For example, How do I report a leaking pipe? How do I escalate the lack of toilet paper? How long has this room been out of action? Do we really need to put the new machine here? As an accessible or present knowledgeable expert, there may be a risk of others assuming IPCSs know everything, particularly if the IPCSs are perceived to be problem solving and proactive. In response, IPCSs may tire of this aspect of their role and reiterate their core purpose and distance themselves from other issues. It could be argued that the IPCSs should facilitate and enable staff to find the solutions, but often it is easier to just do it yourself.

THE POTENTIAL FOR SYNERGY IN WORKING PRACTICE

There are several aspects of healthcare delivery that influence infection prevention and control outcomes, such as product selection, building and design. In addition, numerous aspects of care delivery may enhance value by improving attention to infection prevention and control issues such as cleaning, patient education, patient transport and drug administration.

There are also many aspects of care that could potentially benefit from specialties working synergistically to improve patient outcomes. An example in infection prevention and control is nutrition. Ensuring a patient has adequate nutrition is a fundamental and basic requirement in healthcare. The quality of the food and the food service is a key factor in patient satisfaction.[4]

There are also benefits associated with patient outcome. There is evidence in gastric surgery, for example, that patients who are adequately nourished throughout the surgical journey have improved healthcare outcomes.[5] This includes a reduction in post-operative infection. Nutritional status also influences the immune response of individuals in response to an infection and malnutrition is a risk factor in the acquisition of infection.[6] The nutrition of patients is important in infection prevention and control and ensuring the nutrition of patients is of interest to the IPCS. This is not just to ensure patients do not acquire an infection from the food or food handler, but also to ensure the patient receives adequate nourishment to support immune response, reduce susceptibility to infection and promote recovery from illness. Therefore, it is beneficial if the IPCS champions, supports and facilitates initiatives to improve nutrition.

The same argument applies to many fundamental aspects of care, including sleep and rest, hydration, nausea and vomiting, warmth, stress and anxiety, information, pain control, wound healing, incontinence, prevention of falls, and prevention of pressure sores. The IPCS can, by promoting and supporting other aspects of healthcare delivery with common goals, improve patient outcomes and the value of care delivered. This may be done in many ways and the point will now be illustrated by two examples.

Example one: length of stay

It is well established that the length of time patients stay in healthcare facilities increases their risk of complications such as the acquisition of infection.[7] Generally when this point is made it refers to patients in a hospital bed, but the same principles apply to waiting rooms in clinics or general practitioner surgeries. Therefore, reducing the opportunity time for transmission to take place is beneficial to the patient in reducing his or her risk of infection.

The IPCS can support the process and systems design in clinics, surgeries and hospitals by minimising the impact of infection-related assessment and documentation. This may be as simple as enquiring what information is already known and available and if further assessment is really required. The IPCS can, in addition, support other initiatives from other stakeholders that similarly reduce the time the patient stays in a healthcare facility, such as reducing waiting times for porters, improving early or rapid discharge, or advocating home delivery of prescription drugs.

Example two: diagnostics

It has been established that reducing system delay from initial assessment to final diagnosis and treatment is potentially beneficial to patient outcomes.[8] In part this is reliant on appropriate assessment and the laboratory diagnostic support. The IPCS can support the development of assessment algorithms, ensure staff are clear what tube is required for which test, enquire about all turnaround times of results, ask about delays in specimen deliveries or processing, and use the information to help improve several diagnostic services by highlighting the issues. In acting to optimise the diagnostics associated with infection, by widening the work to include others, the potential benefits are maximised.

UPHOLDING AND MAINTAINING STANDARDS

As mentioned earlier in this chapter, IPCSs often work in many areas of care delivery or other areas supporting delivery. They are therefore in a position to observe care delivery and the standards achieved. While it is not as straightforward as it may appear to determine standards in areas outside your expertise, some aspects of care, such as patients calling out for help or because they are in pain, should prompt IPCSs to make enquiries of the staff. It is not difficult to observe and report issues of safety such as trip hazards, fire risks, lack of security, or lack of privacy and dignity.

Most infection control staff have a background as qualified healthcare workers with a professional responsibility for maintaining and promoting standards of care. Therefore, there is a professional obligation to act on information or observation of poor practice. It is not sufficient to assume that working in a specialty allows staff to ignore or not act on instances that are not within their sphere of control. The expectation is that staff would respond by escalating issues of concern to the appropriate manager and, if this has no effect, to continue to escalate it until it is resolved.

Unfortunately, this is at times problematic for IPCSs. As 'visitors' to an area, they are reliant on the goodwill and cooperation of staff to enable them to identify issues of infection and prevention concern and facilitate the required actions. There is an element of trust involved in a good relationship. This includes openness about a potential lack of knowledge, and the opportunity to ask for help is part of a mutually beneficial and dynamic relationship. To disrupt this by whistleblowing or making complaints may lead to a loss of trust and confidence in the relationship. Therefore, the way this is done is important.

Ultimately, the aim is to highlight and prompt improvement, rather than to irritate and alienate. This is generally easier when there are established and strong relationships with staff in an area. In most instances the role of the IPCS is to reflect back observations (both good and bad) to the appropriate manager or member of staff and to explain the difference between expectations and observed performance. When this is not sufficient, a more formal process of documentation and escalation is required. Sometimes, unfortunately, professional or friendly relationships may be damaged and rebuilding is required. However, if staff are clear that the IPCSs are not habitually trivialising or nitpicking about issues of patient care, then when a concern is raised the IPCSs are more likely to be listened to and their comments valued.

Sometimes, inadvertently, the IPCS becomes aware of an issue that requires action and by highlighting the issue may cause disruption.

Example: causing disruption through highlighting an issue

In a teaching session on basic infection control for delivery drivers in primary care, the IPCS summarised the basic principles of standard precautions and informed the drivers of the risks of blood-borne virus transmission. It was mentioned that any cuts or abrasions on hands should be covered with a plaster. The role of the drivers was to collect and transport used commodes, beds and other patient equipment from patient homes to a centre for cleaning and decontamination prior to reuse. The drivers informed the IPCS that they could not put a plaster on cuts and abrasions, as they had no access to first aid kits, and that they were until that session unaware of the risks to themselves. The manager who is present at the session disputed the need for the provision of first aid kits in vehicles, the drivers called their union representation and a dispute ensued that disrupted the service.

Unfortunately, it is not always possible to avoid this kind of response, particularly in areas that are unfamiliar. Preparation and running through the key elements with managers of the information to be passed on can avoid confusion.

INCREASING INFLUENCE

Three key elements are important in increasing influence and impact:
1. the language and terminology used

2. accurately targeting a consistent message or information
3. understanding the processes required.

Understanding the language to use and the process for making changes or improvements in organisations is important. Each organisation is unique and it is worth making the effort to understand how it functions. It can be very demoralising to fail in efforts to influence change.

A starting point is recognising and understanding the organisational values and objectives. This will indicate the likely priorities and focus of the organisation. If organisational values and objectives, for example, focus on preventing harm and increasing patient satisfaction, then, in explaining the rationale for change, a patient satisfaction and harm-reduction focus in arguments is more likely to be successful in achieving change. Alternatively, in organisations where finance and performance are more important, the language used should include business and finance terminology. However, just because it is not stated in the organisational value statements, do not assume it is not a core value. An example is given in Box 13.1.

BOX 13.1

Problem: Patients get cold walking along a corridor from changing rooms to day surgery and you would like the organisation to provide patients with a warm dressing gown for the journey.

Organisational with primary focus on patient satisfaction
Explanation to organisation: Patients have complained that they get cold in the corridor and it would improve their experience if they were warmed on the journey. If they are warmed they will be less stressed, more comfortable and normothermic. This will increase their satisfaction and reduce their risk of surgical complications.

Organisation with primary focus on value for money and performance
Explanation to organisation: Maintaining a normothermic patient reduces the risk of surgical complications, which thereby reduces length of stay and cost of care. It also increases patient satisfaction with the theatre experience, as they are less stressed and warm, which increases their likelihood of recommending this organisation to others. A cost-benefit analysis indicates that this is cost-effective.

The same approach is useful for communicating with individuals. Using their terminology and understanding their values is crucial. If, for example, you need to influence a staff group with a scientific background who require evidence, the explanation should reflect their language and terminology.

BOX 13.2

Using the same patient warming initiative

Explanation: There is considerable peer-reviewed research evidence that indicates ensuring preoperative and intraoperative normothermia reduces post-operative complications. A number of randomised control trials have demonstrated statistically significant improvements in outcomes.

Understanding the organisational structure is also important, as time may be saved by targeting the message appropriately. This often entails an unravelling of the power rather than managerial structure. In many organisations, although it is clear who is nominally in charge, there is frequently a group of staff who heavily influence the decisions and strategies. Identification of the key influencers and decision makers is an early step in targeting information appropriately and effectively. Time spent on identifying who will be the person who makes the decision saves time in repeating the message to only find you need to speak to someone else.

Determining the required processes, forms, meetings and other organisational controls is also important to success. While this may appear tedious and long winded at times, most processes associated with organisational change have developed to prevent harm or damage and to constrain and manage changes which could disrupt the status quo. It may be difficult to recognise their value while ploughing through the process, but this may be faster than bypassing the system only to encounter failure by not having been through the right process. A fast way of getting this right is to ask someone who has done it successfully before to share his or her knowledge with you.

SUPER SPECIALISTS AND EMBEDDED SPECIALISTS

A particularly effective way to influence change in infection prevention and control is by the development and nurturing of team members with specialist knowledge. This enables staff to understand and speak the language of other specialists in the organisation and, because of their special interest, develop relationships with others with similar interests. This can effectively fast-track conversations and decisions. Examples of this include IPCSs with specialist knowledge or experience in subjects such as decontamination, ventilation, water, environment, blood-borne virus, information technology, and so on.

There are a few IPCSs who now have roles that are predominantly focused on quite narrow aspects of infection prevention and control. An example is an environmental infection control practitioner. The benefits of such roles are manifold, as they have in-depth and current knowledge of the specialty, they can talk the language of engineers, know who to speak to in the organisation about the issues, know how to frame the questions required, understand the answers and are a credible expert. They can also act as a translator of the jargon and act as mediator.

Embedding IPCSs in departments or areas is another way to effectively influence infection prevention and control practice. Specialist areas such as intensive therapy, theatres and dentistry may require particularly focused work to gain engagement and an understanding of the specialty. It can be particularly helpful if the IPCS is working in the area and is part of the team. It is then possible to influence from within, acting as a credible presence. In time the IPCS may be able to utilise the local structures and system within the specialty to promote the infection prevention and control agenda. The embedded IPCS helps to tailor infection prevention and control responses and practice to the constraints of the particular specialty.

There is a potential danger in super specialist and embedded specialist roles that post holders will become so engrossed in the other specialty that they lose sight of their infection prevention and control agenda and become deskilled in the original specialty. To avoid this, job descriptions and plans should make it clear that the super specialist role is one part of the job. Post holders should be supervised and supported to ensure their work output relates to the role expectations.

SELF-EFFICACY

Self-efficacy is an important aspect of increasing influence and value, as frequently the momentum required to influence is dependent on the individual IPCS or the strength and support of the team. Improving self-efficacy can make individuals more effective, which increases their value and in turn boosts their confidence and job satisfaction.

The theory of self-efficacy was first described by Albert Bandura.[9] It is essentially a form of self-confidence in various situations where you have the belief that you are competent to respond appropriately. Bandura[9] described four sources of self-efficacy, as follows.

1. *Performance accomplishments*, which is essentially that by succeeding in experiences you gain confidence in your ability. An example of this could be delivering a lecture or making a presentation; if you do this frequently, you usually gain confidence.

2. *Vicarious experience*, which is that observing people who are similar to you succeeding or failing affects your belief in your own ability to succeed. An example of this would be observing one of your peers competently handling a very difficult conversation with an angry staff member. If they can do it, then you can too.

3. *Verbal persuasion*, which is that people can be persuaded to believe they have the potential or ability to succeed. This could be as simple as a colleague telling you that they believe you are good at something or have the potential to be good at something and that you should try it.

4. *Psychological states*, which is related to people's moods and predisposition that affects their confidence in their ability to succeed. An example of this is people who are in a low mood or are anxious who generally have a more negative perspective on their potential abilities.

Many IPCSs are involved in promoting self-efficacy but are probably unaware of the psychological theory behind it. An example is teaching people to clean their hands and promoting compliance, which is summarised in Table 13.1.

TABLE 13.1 Teaching hand hygiene techniques and promoting compliance

Action	Aspect of self-efficacy theory
Setting up a hand hygiene training session in an appropriate environment that is quiet, the right temperature and where everyone is able to participate easily	Psychological state
Providing an explanation of the value and benefit of hand hygiene	Verbal persuasion
Demonstrating hand hygiene techniques	Vicarious experience
Participants practice and demonstrate techniques	Vicarious experience
Participants get it right and being praised for good technique	Performance accomplishment
Participants repeating the learned technique in practice situations	Performance accomplishment

OTHER WAYS TO BE MORE EFFECTIVE

There are a number of other simple ways to be more effective by managing time and effort. Some brief examples are:

- avoid duplicating the work already done by others
- plan work and set measurable goals
- prioritise
- minimise trivial or time-wasting activities
- simplifying information to ensure comprehension and avoid confusion.

THE VALUE OF INFLUENCE

It is not always easy to measure the value of influence in the workplace. A person in a position of power may have more opportunities than more junior staff to exert influence, and that person's value to the organisation is often reflected by the rewards he or she is offered in salary, status and autonomy.

Infection prevention and control influence may result directly from, for example, education or advice given, or indirectly from, for example, the use of policies and guidelines. The impact of IPCSs is not always immediately obvious and, if successful, it is embedded in practice.

Perhaps the simplest way to assess your own impact is to ask others around you to give you some feedback. There are a number of tools and methods of doing this, but some simple areas to focus on would be as follows.

- Are your views really listened to by others?
- Do people seek your views on issues?
- Have your views and/or actions made a difference?
- Are you asked to collaborate with others?
- Do you receive recognition for your contribution?
- Does the work you do generally achieve positive results?

Another way is to examine the impact and outcomes of work and initiatives. For example, a project to improve invasive device documentation led to a significant reduction in healthcare-associated infections in patients with intravenous devices; or an audit of soap dispensers led to recognition that many were broken and they were subsequently all replaced.

Value and influence may also be perceived as negative. In infection prevention and control it is not uncommon that the requirements are seen as barriers – for example, delaying opening new buildings until they are clean, restricting visiting during outbreaks, removing jackets to wash hands and not eating food in theatres.

While this aspect of the role may not be popular, it is still valuable and it has a positive impact on patient outcomes by contributing to the reduction of healthcare-associated infections.

CONCLUSION

ICPS have opportunities to positively influence practice in healthcare beyond the narrow spectrum of their own specialty. Providing more than the infection prevention and control perspective in a professional and positive way can make a positive contribution to the entire healthcare delivery agenda. This increases the value of their role and optimises their contribution.

REFERENCES

1. Bahamon C, Dwyer J, Buxbaum A. Leading a change process to improve health service delivery. *Bull World Health Organ.* 2006; **84**(8): 658–61.
2. National Audit Office. *Reducing Healthcare Associated Infections in Hospitals in England: report by the Comptroller and Auditor General.* London: The Stationery Office; 2009.
3. Griffiths P, Renz A, Rafferty AM. *The Impact of Organisation and Management Factors on Infection Control in Hospitals: a scoping review.* London: King's College London; 2008.
4. Woodside AG, Frey LL, Daly RT. Linking service quality, customer satisfaction, and behavioural intention. *J Health Care Mark.* 1989; **9**(4): 5–17.
5. Fearon KCH, Luff R. The nutritional management of surgical patients: enhanced recovery after surgery. *Proc Nutr Soc.* 2003; **6**(4): 807–11.
6. Schaible UE, Kaufmann SHE. Malnutrition and infection: complex mechanisms and global impacts. *PLoS Med.* 2007; **4**(5): e115.
7. Delgado-Rodríguez M, Bueno-Cavanillas A, López-Gigosos R, *et al.* Hospital stay length as an effect modifier of other risk factors for nosocomial infection. *Eur J Epidemiol.* 1990; **6**(1): 34–9.
8. Olesen F, Hansen RP, Vedsted P. Delay in diagnosis: the experience in Denmark. *Br J Cancer.* 2009; 101(Suppl. 2): S5–8.
9. Bandura A. *Self-efficacy: the exercise of control.* New York, NY: WH Freeman; 1997.

CHAPTER 14

The use of marketing in infection prevention and control

....

Annette Jeanes

Marketing is used widely in everyday life. This chapter will introduce simple marketing concepts and explain how these can be applied in infection prevention and control.

MARKETING

Marketing is the process through which products, ideas or behaviours are promoted to a customer or audience. This includes market research and advertising, and it is used widely to sell or influence choices. The basic elements are the 4 Ps of marketing: Product, Price, Place and Promotion. This may be expanded to the 7 Ps by adding People, Process and Physical evidence.

These elements of marketing are summarised briefly here.

1. **Product**: to be marketable the product should be something that people will want or need.
2. **Price**: the product should be value for money and affordable, or the price people are willing to pay. It may be priced to be extremely expensive and this may increase the desirability.
3. **Place**: the product should be accessible, in the right or convenient place and at the right time for the user or purchaser.
4. **Promotion**: this is the communication to the customer about the product and includes advertising; promotion may also include straplines and images.

5. **People** – this generally applies to the people promoting and or selling the product. It could also include the endorsement of reputable experts.

6. **Process**: this relates to how the product is delivered to the customer. This includes how the product comes to the customer's attention, the way it is selected and ordered, and how it is delivered.

7. **Physical evidence**: this relates to feedback from customers and evidence about the product, the process, the price and the people involved. This information is used to modify the product, promotion, price, process, and so forth, but also to demonstrate to others that the product is being used and acquired by others. An example would be: '8 out of 10 people use ...'.

There are so many examples of marketing in healthcare that you are probably barely aware of it most of the time. Every product purchased and used is marketed to some degree as part of the procurement process. This includes the flooring of a healthcare facility, the paint on the walls, the bulbs in the lights, the water in the taps, the disposable gloves, the uniforms and more.

TABLE 14.1 Examples of the 7 Ps in use

Element	Example
Product	Safety-engineered phlebotomy kit
Price	Preferably the same price or less than non-safety devices
Place	Easily accessible for phlebotomists (i.e. on their standard workstation set-up)
Promotion	Clear labelling and logo; posters, education and information about preventing sharps injury
People	Occupational health staff, sales representatives
Process	Introduction of product to users, staff who order it and training in how to use the product safely
Physical evidence	Feedback from users and rates of sharps injuries

The techniques used to market products range from the obvious shouting of a market trader to the more subtle or subliminal advertising campaigns. Many companies employ highly paid and highly skilled experts in marketing. Usually the marketers have a vested interest in the success of the product and the success of the marketing strategy. It is unusual for established organisations and institutions to ignore the value of marketing, as it creates and nurtures the brand and contributes to the success, value and sustainability of the products produced. Marketing and the associated issues of image, profile, market share and profit are closely linked in many companies.

Unfortunately, in healthcare, marketing is often not perceived to be a high priority and may be particularly poorly resourced at a local level. Consequently, in infection prevention and control, practitioners frequently resort to a 'do it yourself' methodology, which can sometimes be brilliant but is often not, and which can appear amateurish in comparison with professional campaigns.

At a national level, marketing is frequently used to change health-related behaviours. This is usually referred to as social marketing.

SOCIAL MARKETING

Social marketing uses marketing techniques to change or influence behaviours for the good of all.[1] Essentially, it is an approach aimed at selling attitudes, behaviours and ideas. It is used extensively in healthcare. Examples of social marketing are:

- anti-smoking campaigns
- anti-alcohol campaigns
- breast cancer screening
- condom use promotion.

Social marketing varies from standard marketing in several ways. While there is generally a financial benefit in promoting a physical product for profit, in social marketing the benefit is accrued and measured by the effect on behaviours and attitudes. Social marketing is often linked to public policies and strategies that may be linked to a resource to fund the marketing. The audience may be very wide and variable. Social marketing may also be aimed at influencing policymakers and it may seek to alter social and cultural norms. Examples of this include campaigns about the disabled and racism. In these instances, different organisations with similar aims will collaborate to support these marketing campaigns.

The 4 Ps are used, but as a starting point often the campaigns and techniques attempt to increase awareness that there is a problem. The product then becomes the solution. An example would be: 'smoking can cause lung cancer; therefore, the solution is to stop smoking'.

In social marketing, hard-hitting images and messages may be used when previous, softer messages have not worked on some of the target audience. Advertising relating to preventing road traffic accidents is a good example of progressively hard-hitting campaigns. Initially, these aimed at increasing alertness to traffic when crossing a road and at reducing speed. Later campaigns were progressively more explicit for some target audiences; in some there were images of death and dying. The product is about road safety but the method of delivering the message is to frighten and to make people identify with the victims. Similar approaches are used in anti-smoking and anti-hunting campaigns.

The price element associated with social marketing is usually the benefit gained by individuals or society, but it can deliver public savings such as a reduction in patients admitted following road traffic accidents or a reduction in patients dying of lung cancer. Therefore, the saving and benefit is largely for society as a whole.

The place of the product in social marketing may relate to how consumers get help or advice or how the message reaches the target audience. This process requires a clear understanding of who are the target audience and how likely they are to use or have contact with various media formats. It would be ineffective to promote the value of a website to people with no access to the Internet, for example. The placement of the product or message is heavily dependent on understanding the target audience. This may result in numerous methods of product placement, including posters, television adverts, Internet messages, newspaper and magazines, food wrappers, and so on.

Social marketing also has to contend with the fatigue of the audience, when they eventually ignore and grow bored with the message being promoted. In campaigns funded by industries selling products, the sale of the product can then generate more resource for marketing and the campaign is subsequently changed and updated. In social marketing, as a problem becomes less of an issue or an issue less of a problem, funding may become scarce and campaigns may not be refreshed regularly – particularly as there is competition for other issues and causes.

MARKETING CAMPAIGNS

Many in infection prevention and control will be motivated to run a campaign or launch an initiative or promote an idea, concept or behaviour. This could be related to the service provided or to a particular initiative. To do this effectively you may decide to develop a marketing campaign. There are numerous detailed examples of marketing campaigns on the Internet. This section provides a short guide that briefly summarises how to set up and run a marketing campaign.

The first step is to understand why you are doing it. What is the purpose of your campaign? If you are not clear, then others will not be clear either.

Associated with the purpose, you need to decide who your campaign or initiative is aimed at. Who are you marketing to? This may include children, adults, families, healthcare workers, general public, non-English speakers, and so on. The characteristics of the target audience will influence your approach, the ideas you develop, the language you use and the method of communication you select.

Next are the budget and/or resource. If this venture is likely to require significant resource then you may need to develop a business case or proposal for funding. In some organisations this sort of budget is included in the departmental running cost. You may have to decide if sponsorship is an option. Resource is not just about the money. It is also about the available talent and enthusiasm and the use of facilities or resource (e.g. photocopiers). You may have to market your proposal to potential marketing recruits (colleagues) or the people responsible for the resources you hope or plan to use.

Then you need to decide on a strategy and plan. This will be constrained by the resource and time you have available. Key elements to include are not only how will you do it and who will you aim it at, but also:

- What are your targets or goals?
- How will you measure success?
- What is your backup plan if your efforts fail or falter?
- What are the risks?

It is essential that you are clear and realistic about your focus and aspiration, as to be too ambitious with poorly thought-out ideas will mean you are less likely to succeed. In addition, test your underlying assumptions and your propositions to ensure they are robust. A popular method is to create a focus group to test these and ensure others agree with you and your approach.

Box 14.1 shows an example from a hand hygiene compliance improvement campaign.

In response to feedback from staff and patient groups, the campaign was modified to focus on how easy it could be to transmit infection. The patients in particular were keen to ensure all healthcare workers understood that they could pass on infections by not cleaning hands. It was agreed that this was unacceptable and avoidable. This led to a campaign idea: 'Don't be the one to pass it on', which was aimed at provoking an emotional response from staff and the public.

How you then develop your initiative or campaign may vary, but a simple, engaging and consistent approach may be more successful than one that confuses or alienates. A slogan or strapline is often used but is not essential, although it is helpful if you produce something that is memorable.

There must be a plan for a launch and a communication strategy. This is often an opportunity for leaders in an organisation to give a supportive statement, and to have a picture taken promoting the campaign or project. Although this may seem

---

BOX 14.1 Hand hygiene compliance improvement campaign

Assumptions

- Everyone is potentially at fault
- We need to change behaviour and attitudes
- Parallels exist between hand hygiene and other public health campaigns that have been tackled successfully
- Everyone needs to talk openly about the importance of hand hygiene
- Raising awareness will lead to greater personal responsibility

Propositions

- Failure of staff to clean their hands is unacceptable, irresponsible and negligent
- The public should not be afraid to challenge staff about hand hygiene

---

like the end of the work, it is important that the people involved are fully briefed and are clear about what is going to happen. Although by this point you may be tired of the message yourself, it is important to ensure it is repeated at every opportunity.

An evaluation of the campaign is useful in understanding what went well and what could be improved in a subsequent campaign. This could be through a simple questionnaire, interviews or measuring product uptake (e.g. soap, for hand hygiene).

The following questions summarise these basic elements of a marketing campaign:

- What is the purpose of your marketing?
- What are your targets and goals?
- Who is the target audience and what are their characteristics?
- What budget or resources are available?
- What is the timescale?
- What is your idea/s or initiative?
- What is your strategy and plan?
- Do you have a contingency plan?
- Have you tested your marketing propositions and assumptions?
- Have you modified your campaign ideas in response to feedback?
- What is your communication and launch plan?
- What was learned from the evaluation?

FINALLY

Key aspects of the work of infection prevention and control practitioners is to pro-mote and change behaviours, to introduce new products and to improve practice. Marketing is therefore a useful tool. The basics of marketing methods are simple and can be adapted; a good starting point is to reflect on how you market yourself and your services.

REFERENCE

1. Kotler P, Zaltman G. Social marketing: an approach to planned social change. *J Mark.* 1971; **35**(3): 3–12.

CHAPTER 15

Patient and healthcare worker empowerment

....

Maryanne McGuckin

Fifteen years ago when my colleagues and I introduced the concept of empowering patients to ask their healthcare workers (HCWs) to wash their hands as a way to increase hand hygiene (HH) compliance, there was a great deal of doubt that this would be possible. Our programme, Partners in Your Care,[1] was embraced by many, and yet there was some scepticism that unfortunately continues among some colleagues, despite the evidence for success. Those who do not fully embrace this concept are looking for the double-blind controlled study as proof of efficacy, rather than alternative methods for testing such as developing and evaluating pilot programmes with the professionals most likely to know the environment in which the programmes will be applied: the HCW and specifically the infection preventionist. Doubters continue their trend of identifying barriers to patient and HCW empowerment rather than keeping their focus patient centred. As a pioneer of this concept, and the author of over a dozen peer-reviewed articles in which patient empowerment was studied using a standardised quantitative measurement model, there is evidence to support patient empowerment in our HH programmes. It is time for us to stop looking for reasons why patient empowerment may not work and to encourage creative programmes and share our successes. There will always be patients and HCWs who will not embrace the concept of patient empowerment, just as there are still HCWs who do not embrace sanitiser usage or the World Health Organization's (WHO) Five Moments for Hand Hygiene, but that should not be a reason for not including patient empowerment in our (HH) programmes. We would not think of stopping the use of sanitiser until we find out the psychological or social issues of why some HCWs are not using sanitiser or following the five moments. We must focus on the pros of patient empowerment and not the cons. Waiting for the perfect study that will say patient empowerment and HH compliance works or does not work will not change the fact that our patients are demanding to be empowered and to participate in their care, and it is our responsibility as HCWs to provide them with skills and knowledge to be empowered. In addition, several regulatory organisations are recommending, and for some rewarding, patient participation. As the author of a recent review of patient empowerment and HH, there is evidence that, in principle, patients are willing to be empowered. However, there is variation in the actual number of patients who practise empowerment for HH, ranging from 5% to 80%. A key factor driving lower numbers is the lack of having an intervention using programmes that include education, measurement, feedback and explicit permission from HCWs to patients to be empowered.[2]

Therefore, the objective of this chapter is to help the infection preventionist develop programmes that empower both HCWs and patients so that they become more comfortable in their roles. Barriers will be presented as a way for you to be aware of them and should not be used as reasons for not including patient empowerment in your programmes. We can no longer wait for that perfect study that identifies all barriers, and while we wait, cast doubt among HCWs. Yes, it is time to embrace patient empowerment, as it is the right thing to do for patient safety.

INTRODUCTION

When you need hospital care, it's comforting to know that you've chosen a good hospital and a good doctor who will look out for your welfare. However, as healthcare providers, we should not expect that patients will just lie back and wait to get better. Patients and HCWs have definite rights and responsibilities for the delivery and outcome of care. As early as 1977, WHO advocated that patients participate in their healthcare.[3] We now know that empowering both HCW and patient can have a significant effect on the prevention of healthcare-associated infections (HCAIs).[4] Empowerment has been defined as a process in which patients understand their opportunity to contribute, and are given the knowledge and skills by their healthcare provider and other educational sources to perform a task in an environment that recognises community and cultural differences and encourages patient participation.[2]

You will notice that whenever possible, I prefer using the term empowerment and not softer terms such as patient involvement, patient participation, and patient engagement. Although these alternative terms have been used in the hope that patients would be more likely to feel safer with these words, one needs to realise that in order to participate, be involved or be engaged, one first needs to be empowered with knowledge, skills and, most important, an environment that encourages their involvement.

WILLINGNESS OF PATIENTS TO BE EMPOWERED

In 2004, WHO launched the World Alliance for Patient Safety to raise awareness and political commitment to improve the safety of care in all its member states.[5] A specific area of work, Patients for Patient Safety, was designed to ensure that the wisdom of patients, families, consumers, and citizens, in both developed and developing countries, is central in shaping the work of the alliance.

The extent to which patients wish to be empowered is still a matter of debate, as I explained in the opening section. For example, Longtin *et al.*[6] discussed the reasons why patients would not ask about HH, based on an open questionnaire given to 194 patients. The main reasons were the perception that caregivers already know (or should know) when to perform HH, the belief that asking about HH is not part of the patient's role, and a feeling of embarrassment or awkwardness associated with asking about HH. However, we must realise that an important part of empowerment is to first give knowledge. Without this knowledge, one would expect a patient to not see the value of participation. This is supported by a 2010 study in Sweden, looking at patients' understanding of patient participation. The study found that patients reported and described participation mainly as sharing knowledge and sharing respect. They wanted to have knowledge rather than just being informed, and they wanted to interact with health professionals, rather than merely partaking in decision making.[7] Another survey of over 2000 consumers found that 91% thought they could prevent medical errors occurring in hospitals, and 98% thought that hospitals should educate patients in this regard.[8] One can conclude from these findings that consumers understand they can make a difference in preventing errors but still have their own perceived ideas of what are the most important patient safety errors. It is the HCW's role to give this knowledge and permission to participate. Reflection 15.1 is an example of how one HCW learned what advocacy means.

REFLECTION 15.1 Daughter, healthcare worker and advocate[10]

I have been a healthcare professional for more than 25 years, and now I am also a healthcare patient advocate. Throughout my nursing career, I always acted as an advocate for my patients. That often meant going against the usual routine within the work environment and trying new care practices to protect patients.

Then my father developed pneumonia due to resistant bacteria called meticillin-resistant *Staphylococcus aureus* (MRSA) infection. He almost died because of a lack of basic infection control practices in the hospital where he was treated. That is when the need for a different kind of advocacy hit closer to home. Until that time, I was always advocating for safe care, but I was not specifically focused on preventing infections.

While my Dad was hospitalised, I began to see what hospital care was like from a patient's perspective. Basic infection control practices were lacking. No one performed the patient care practices that are designed to prevent pneumonia, such as oral care and elevating the head of the bed.

The most important failure was the lack of hand washing. We contacted the infection control department as well as the chief nurse and were told that, 'We are aware of the problems and are working on them.' I realised that asking about hand washing was not going to make an impact on patient care, because there were so many offenders. Instead, I placed a sign on the door to my Dad's hospital room that said, 'Wash hands'. At this point, I needed no additional evidence that it is the responsibility of an advocate (often a family member) to monitor infection control practices together with the healthcare team and take direct action to protect a loved one's health and safety in the hospital.

A patient's willingness to be empowered is dependent on having gathered enough information, understanding how to use the information, and being convinced that this knowledge gives them shared responsibility with their HCWs. However, in their review of materials given to patients to empower them, Coulter and colleagues[9] found that relevant information was often omitted, many doctors adopted a patronising tone, and few actively promoted a shared approach. Studies have also shown that patients prefer information that is specific, given by their HCWs, and printed for use as prompt sheets if necessary. How many of the steps outlined in Reflection 15.2 do you or your colleagues include in your patient empowerment programmes?

REFLECTION 15.2 What patients need is empathy and empowerment (courtesy of Kerry O'Connell, infected patient and advocate)[10]

- Tell us how we [the patients] can be empowered to take an active part in our care
- Always tell the patient what organism he has been blessed with
- Tell the patient the most likely ways he contracted his infection
- Lay out in detail the good, the bad and the ugly prognosis
- Spend time with patients in the isolation ward (the loneliest place on earth)
- Give us some solid clues on how to prevent this next time
- Learn to express genuine remorse
- Never ever send survey form letters to known victims
- Love thy infected patient (even the very difficult ones)

In addition to having knowledge as part of empowerment, patients also need skills, and an important one is what we call self-efficacy. Although there are several components of the concept of self-efficacy, verbal persuasion is probably the most relevant to a patient being empowered. Verbal persuasion affects an individual's perceived ability to believe that he or she can in fact be empowered.[11] Another concept that affects a patient's willingness to be empowered is health literacy, which is the ability to understand health information and to use that information to make good decisions about health and medical care. Health literacy is fundamental to patient empowerment.[12]

In summary, a patient's willingness to be involved, empowered or engaged is dependent on the overall environment of the organisation and its attitudes toward patient safety and patient involvement.

APPLICATION TO INFECTION CONTROL

In studies undertaken in the United States and the United Kingdom, McGuckin and colleagues[1,13,14] reported on the willingness of patients to be empowered and involved in HH by asking their HCWs to clean their hands. They documented that 80%–90% of patients will agree to ask in principle, but the percentage of those who actually asked their HCW is slightly lower, at 60%–70%. This was further reinforced by the findings of the evaluation of the pilot testing of the National Patient Safety Agency of England's Clean Your Hands campaign.[15] They reported that the majority of patients believed the public should be involved in helping staff increase their HH compliance.

A survey of consumers on their attitudes about HH found that four out of five consumers said they would ask their HCW, 'Did you wash/sanitise your hands?' if their HCW educated them on the importance of HH.[16] Longitin and colleagues[17] presented a conceptual model of patient empowerment looking at factors of knowledge and applicability to patient safety. For infection control, especially HH, they believe that patients can be a source of education to staff. They state, 'organizing a campaign that encourages patients to ask HCWs about HH would draw HCWs attention to its importance and raise their adherence without patients having to intervene.'[17]

WILLINGNESS OF HEALTHCARE WORKERS TO BE EMPOWERED

In patient empowerment, the HCW strives to promote and enhance the patient's abilities to feel in control of his or her health. Education and decision aides – for example, leaflets, computer programs, interactive videos, websites and group presentations – are useful to healthcare providers in the process of empowering patients.[18] The aim of these tools is to help patients reflect on and identify their own skills and needs and realise that these skills will have a benefit in their lives.[19] However, the healthcare professional's perceptions of patient knowledge influence how patients are involved in decision making and being empowered. Patients who can communicate health knowledge involve themselves in ways that are perceived as beneficial, but patients who lack that ability may be active and engaged but are excluded from decision making or being empowered. By being aware of that bias, healthcare professionals may be able to be more effective in empowering all patients.[20]

A review of patient engagement and what works by Coulter[21] states that (a) contrary to popular belief there is a great deal of published evidence on the likely effectiveness of patient engagement strategies and (b) there is a compelling case for reviewing and, where necessary, adapting healthcare delivery and practice styles to enable active engagement of patients in planning and shaping their healthcare. The message is very clear that a significant part of patient empowerment is HCW empowerment and the HCW's role in giving patients explicit help in becoming involved. Yvonne Birks and colleagues[22] carried out a series of studies to examine how patients and their representatives might promote their own safety in healthcare and identified the following four factors as important to patient empowerment.

1. Patients are likely to need the support of healthcare professionals to participate in contributing to safer healthcare initiatives.
2. Nurses are well placed to support patients to voice concerns about the safety of their care.

3. Patients may feel reluctant to express concern where nursing staff are perceived to be unreceptive to concerns.

4. Organisations should support nursing staff to enable patient involvement in patient safety in a number of ways.

Similar findings were reported in 2007 when WHO conducted a two-part survey on patient empowerment to gain further knowledge and to incorporate geographically and culturally diverse perspectives related to empowerment into the final version of the *WHO Guidelines for Hand Hygiene in Healthcare*.[2] One of the key findings was that HCWs' active encouragement to the patient to remind HCWs about HH had a significant impact on a patient's willingness to be empowered.

The issue remains on the best approach to empower HCWs so that they in turn can empower their patients. There are three prerequisites that HCWs require if they are expected to help patients be seen as able to be empowered.[23] These are (1) a workplace that promotes empowerment; (2) a personal belief that patients, regardless of their knowledge of healthcare issues, can be empowered; and (3) acknowledgement that the relationship and communication of HCWs with patients can be powerful and result in trust and encouragement to be proactive in their role as an advocate for patient safety. It is important to remember that a HCW cannot create personal empowerment in another individual. However, the partnership of HCWs and patients can facilitate or bring about a sense of being able to be empowered. If patients are given knowledge and resources in an environment of mutual respect and support, then a facilitating environment for empowerment will develop.

APPLICATION TO INFECTION CONTROL

There are many opportunities for HCWs to empower their patients on a daily basis about clinical issues such as diabetes control, hypertension medication and nutrition. Although these are empowerment concepts, HCWs have often seen them more as education tools as opposed to concepts aimed at underpinning the facilitation of empowerment. However, when one considers infection prevention and control, the most frequently studied example of patient empowerment relates to HH improvement, and here lies the task of making sure the HCW is first empowered. Patient and HCW empowerment programmes for HH should be part of any basic multimodal HH improvement strategy. The strategy proposed by WHO to implement the Guidelines on Hand Hygiene includes five key elements and should be reviewed before one considers patient empowerment.[2,4] The foundation of the strategy must be ownership, accountability and shared responsibility. Just as patients need to be part of the development of materials and programmes for patients, HCWs must see that they have a shared responsibility and ownership in the development of patient-empowerment programmes. For example, one cannot start a programme of encouraging patients to ask their HCWs to wash or sanitise their hands unless there has been buy-in from key stakeholders and input from HCWs into the programme. The value of involving HCWs has been supported by the work of Longtin *et al.*[24] in a survey of 277 HCWs on their perception of patients asking them about HH. They found that 29% did not support the idea of being reminded by patients to perform HH – even though 74% of respondents said they believed that patients could help prevent HCAIs. The researchers also found that 44% of respondents said they would feel guilty if patients discovered they skipped HH, and 43% said they would feel ashamed to disclose such a fact. This survey gives us some important information on how HCWs may believe that an empowered patient is important to patient safety, but lacking a personal belief that they should be empowered can result in a belief that it is not the patient's role to ask about HH.

Empowerment programmes for infection control and specifically for HH can be categorised into educational (including Internet), motivational (reminders and posters), and role-modelling within the context of a multimodal approach. The WHO Guidelines[2] and McGuckin and Govednik[25] provide an excellent overview of the research for each of these categories and should be reviewed before deciding on a specific process. It is essential that an evaluation component be part of all empowerment programmes.

OVERCOMING BARRIERS TO EMPOWERMENT

There are several different theories from various disciplines that provide insight into the potential barriers to patient empowerment in healthcare. These theories include cognitive, behavioural, social marketing and organisational theories that may be valuable when considering barriers to be overcome, or a strategy to involve and engage patients.[26] It is important to remember that the foundation of an empowerment programme is ownership and shared responsibility. Therefore, barriers are better addressed if we acknowledge different views on patient empowerment and deal with them in the context of an organisation, culture or community. The UK National Patient Safety Agency surveyed the public, inpatients and HCWs – particularly front-line clinical staff and infection control nurses – in five acute care hospitals to determine whether they agreed on a greater level of involvement. A key finding was that most HCWs surveyed (71%) said that HCAIs could be reduced to a greater or lesser degree if patients asked HCWs if they had cleaned their hands before touching them.[27] Following publication of the findings of this work in the academic press, a follow-up letter to the editor from a HCW presenting details following her hospitalisation presents yet another barrier to empowerment. She voices concern that we may be moving the responsibility of HH from HCW to patient and that not all patients want and can be empowered.[28] Here we see the continued focus on barriers and reasons why empowerment will not work, rather than developing programmes for high-dependency patients. For example, a study in an intensive care unit in the United States used voice prompts developed by administrative and medical leadership reminding HCWs to wash or sanitise their hands, and the prompts were played from the nursing stations. In this model, the voice prompts served as the advocate for the non-communicative patients. They reported a significant increase in HH compliance using this model.[29] One of the hand-washing pioneers, Semmelweiss, never gave up and we cannot give up on encouraging patient empowerment. Reflection 15.3 addresses why we must face each barrier with a solution and that solution can no longer be 'why it will not work'.

REFLECTION 15.3 Guilt to empowerment[10]

My mother was a registered nurse. She walked daily for exercise, enjoyed gardening, and was a very active 70-year-old woman. So what went wrong?

On Thanksgiving (25 November 2004, 6 weeks after her surgery), my mother began complaining of nausea. She didn't have fever, diarrhoea or vomiting, so I thought she might have food poisoning. I called her surgeon, who didn't seem alarmed. He never suggested that I should take my mother to a hospital, but the next morning, I took her to the hospital myself. She died there 10 hours later from a massive infection.

This began my search to find out what went wrong. How had she acquired that infection? How could it have been prevented? It was only after I requested her autopsy report that I learned the results from her laboratory culture. It was an MRSA infection. Looking back at my mother's ordeal, I now realise many things that would have been helpful to know and steps that could have been taken to prevent the tragedy of her untimely death. Like most people, we assumed that reputable hospitals take every precaution necessary to ensure that their patients are cared for in a safe and sanitary way. After our mother's death, we found that this is not always the case.

In retrospect, I now understand what I should have been told by the HCWs to reduce her risk of MRSA infection. Knowing what I know now about the dangers of HCAIs after surgery, particularly MRSA, I would have insisted that greater precautions be taken to ensure that proper sterile techniques were used during each step of her care. We would have insisted that each person entering my mother's hospital room would be required to wash or sanitise his or her hands and that all equipment in my mother's hospital room be adequately disinfected. Knowledge is power, and unfortunately I wish that I had the knowledge then, so that I could have protected my mother from the thing she feared the most: a hospital error.

TRENDING: EASY ACCESS TO INFORMATION AND SOCIAL MEDIA

Healthcare social media can be defined as the interactive engagement through use of electronic platform(s) for the multidirectional exchange of user-generated information, knowledge, data and wisdom including anecdotal experiences among patients, their families, healthcare professionals, health researchers and healthcare administrators.[30] Advocates of the use of social media in healthcare suggest that these applications allow for personalisation and participation – key elements that make them highly effective.[31] Content can be tailored to the priorities of the users, and the collaborative nature of social media allows for a meaningful contribution from all user groups. Clearly these qualities are ideal for empowering our patients, with capabilities of doing so in real time, giving them the knowledge and skills they need to be active participants in their care.

The evidence is growing in support of this new trend. A study in the United Kingdom found 51% of adults go online for health tips, compared with 20% going to a doctor for advice.[32] Similar results were found in the United States: 59% of adults in the United States say they have looked online for health information in the past year.[33] In another study, 52% of US 'smartphone' (phones with Internet capability) owners gather health information on their phones. Cell phone owners who are Latino or African American, are between the ages of 18 and 49, or hold a college degree are also more likely to gather health information this way.[34] Although not all consumers have Internet access or use it to seek health information, it is clearly one of the primary modes of information sharing. These studies document the potential of online communities, online peer groups, and social networks can have on an individual consumer's decision. By 2012, 24% of respondents to a US survey reported posting a health experience or update to a social network; 16% posted reviews of medications or treatments of doctors or insurers.[35] We anticipate the numbers will increase with time. Access to the Internet, use of smartphones (meaning access all the time), and information-seeking activity on health experiences might be the next source for momentum in our empowerment direction. How will HCWs who participate in consumer peer networks allow for consumers to freely share their experiences while maintaining a standard of quality? These are the challenges we face as consumers are seeking information more from the Internet than from qualified professionals.

Will patient satisfaction – or, how we like to say, 'happy patients, good outcomes' – help us empower patients through social media and make them participate in their care? Is patient satisfaction really patient safety and empowerment, or is it a way for hospitals to generate revenue by getting good scores on their surveys and therefore additional revenue. There is, however, the potential to adopt these programmes for HH and empowerment. Giving patients an opportunity to voice a complaint at the time HH does not occur, through some form of social media device, and get a response can be a surrogate for empowerment and at the same time generate compliance data.

AWARENESS, ENGAGEMENT AND INTENTION

There is no doubt that both consumers and patients are aware of this silent epidemic of HCAIs, but how aware are they that the single most important factor in preventing HCAIs is HH and that compliance is still less than 50% of the time among HCWs? Do we tell our patients this fact when they are admitted as a way to engage them? No, but we are eager to survey them on their intention on asking their HCW to sanitise his or her hands and then we are surprised to find out that patients think this is being done and why should they need to be concerned. There lies the fault. We need more transparency about HH compliance rates. I am sure if we first told patients the facts, their responses would be different.

You will recall in the reflections, the message was always the same: 'if only I knew'. A recent study of adult patients who had HCAI and were placed in contact precautions were surveyed about their willingness to learn about multidrug-resistant organisms and HCAIs and their preferred ways of education about multidrug-resistant organism HCAIs. Ninety-eight per cent of patients thought that their involvement in learning about multidrug-resistant organisms was very important or important. Most of the patients thought that receiving information about multidrug-resistant organisms would probably or definitely help them to make choices that would improve their healthcare. The authors concluded that patient preferences must be incorporated into education to increase engagement for prevention of HCAIs.[36] Similar research was done with consumers and their intention to use public reports of HCAIs in their decision to choose a doctor or hospital.

The authors found that only 36% of consumers knew their states had reports (awareness), of which only 12% looked up the report (engagement), and only 52% had intention of using the reports in the future.[37] In 2012, the Agency for Healthcare Research and Quality, as part of their programme Closing the Quality Gap, states that patient and families are just not aware that quality information is available.[38]

Patient empowerment can take on many forms, depending on the culture, environment and resources, but we must keep in mind that making our patients aware of the need to ask and to give permission will remove barriers.

ACKNOWLEDGEMENTS

I wish to thank Ms Kyan Chuong, library science graduate student from Drexel University and the University of Pennsylvania, Philadelphia, for her assistance in the literature review process, and Mr John Govednik, MS, Research Associate/Education Coordinator for McGuckin Methods International, for his assistance in the review and editing of the manuscript.

REFERENCES

1. McGuckin M, Waterman R, Porten L, *et al*. Patient education model for increasing handwashing compliance. *Am J Infect Control*. 1999; **27**(4): 309–14.
2. World Health Organization (WHO). *The WHO Guidelines on Hand Hygiene in Health Care*. Geneva: WHO; 2009.
3. Bissell P, May CR, Noyce PR. From compliance to concordance: barriers to accomplishing a re-framed model of health care interactions. *Soc Sci Med*. 2004; **58**(4): 851–62.
4. McGuckin M, Storr J, Longtin Y, *et al*. Patient empowerment and multimodal hand hygiene promotion: a win-win strategy. *Am J Med Qual*. 2011; **26**(1): 10–17.
5. World Health Organization. *Patient Safety: World Alliance for Patient Safety. The launch of the World Alliance for Patient Safety, Washington DC, USA – 27 October 2004*. Geneva: World Health Organization; 2004. Available at: www.who.int/patientsafety/worldalliance/en/ (accessed 29 October 2013).
6. Longtin Y, Sax H, Allegranzai B, *et al*. Patients' beliefs and perceptions of their participation to increase staff compliance with hand hygiene. *Infect Control Hosp Epidemiol*. 2009; **30**(9): 830–9.
7. Eldh AC, Ekman I, Ehnfors M. A comparison of the concept of patient participation and patients' descriptions as related to healthcare definitions. *Int J Nurs Terminol Classif*. 2010; **21**(1): 21–32.
8. Waterman AD, Gallagher TH, Garbutt J, *et al*. Brief report: hospitalized patients' attitudes about and participation in error prevention. *J Gen Intern Med*. 2006; **21**(4): 367–70.
9. Coulter A, Entwistle V, Gilbert D. Sharing decisions with patients: is the information good enough? *BMJ*. 1999; **318**(7179): 318–22.
10. McGuckin M, Goldfarb T. *The Patient Survival Guide: 8 simple solutions to prevent hospital and healthcare associated infections*. New York, NY: Demos Medical Publishing; 2012.

11. Coulter A, Ellins J. Effectiveness of strategies for informing, educating, and involving patients. *BMJ.* 2007; **335**(7609): 24–7.
12. Bandura A. *Social Foundations of Thought and Action.* Englewood Cliffs, NJ: Prentice Hall; 1977.
13. McGuckin M, Waterman R, Storr J, *et al.* Evaluation of a patient-empowering hand hygiene programme in the UK. *J Hosp Infect.* 2001; **48**(3): 222–7.
14. McGuckin M, Taylor A, Martin V, *et al.* Evaluation of a patient education model for increasing hand hygiene compliance in an inpatient rehabilitation unit. *Am J Infect Control.* 2004; **32**(4): 235–8.
15. Rande J, Clarke M, Storr J. Hand hygiene compliance in healthcare workers. *Am J Hosp Infect.* 2006; **64**(3): 205–9.
16. McGuckin M, Waterman R, Shubin A. Consumer attitudes about health care-acquired infections and hand hygiene. *Am J Med Qual.* 2006; **21**(5): 342–6.
17. Longtin Y, Sax H, Leape L, *et al.* Patient participation: current knowledge and applicability to patient safety. *Mayo Clin Proc.* 2010; **85**(1): 53–62.
18. Holmström I, Röing M. The relation between patient-centeredness and patient empowerment: a discussion on concepts. *Patient Educ Couns.* 2010; **79**(2): 167–72.
19. Ellis-Stoll CC, Popkess-Vawter S. A concept analysis on the process of empowerment. *ANS Adv Nurs Sci.* 1998; **21**(2): 62–8.
20. Heldal F, Steinsbekk A. Norwegian healthcare professionals' perceptions of patient knowledge and involvement as basis for decision making in hematology. *Oncol Nurs Forum.* 2009; **36**(2): E93–8.
21. Coulter A. Patient engagement – what works? *J Ambul Care Manage.* 2012; **35**(2): 80–9.
22. Birks Y, Hall J, McCaughan D, *et al.* Promoting patient involvement in safety initiatives. *Nurs Manag (Harrow).* 2011; **18**(1): 16–20.
23. Manojlovich M. Power and empowerment in nursing: looking backward to inform the future. *Online J Issues Nurs.* 2007; **12**(1): 2.
24. Longtin Y, Farquet N, Gayet-Ageron A, *et al.* Caregivers' perceptions of patients as reminders to improve hand hygiene. *Arch Intern Med.* 2012; **172**(19): 1516–17.
25. McGuckin M, Govednik J. Patient empowerment and hand hygiene, 1997–2012. *J Hosp Infect.* 2013; **84**(3): 191–9.
26. Howe A. Can the patient be on our team? An operational approach to patient involvement in interprofessional approaches to safe care. *J Interprof Care.* 2006; **20**(5): 527–34.
27. Pittet D, Panesar S, Wilson K, *et al.* Involving the patient to ask about hospital hand hygiene: a National Patient Safety Agency feasibility study. *J Hosp Infect.* 2011; **77**: 299–303.
28. Hill D. Hand hygiene: are we trying to make the patient the fail-safe system? *J Hosp Infect.* 2011; **79**(4): 381–2.
29. McGuckin M, Shubin A, McBride P, *et al.* The effect of random voice hand hygiene messages delivered by medical, nursing, and infection control staff on hand hygiene compliance in intensive care. *Am J Infect Control.* 206; **34**(3): 673–5.
30. Schein R, Wilson K, Keelen J. *Literature Review on Effectiveness of the Use of Social Media: a report for Peel Public Health.* Brampton, ON: Peel Public Health; 2010.
31. Centers for Disease Control and Prevention (US). *Social Media Toolkit.* Atlanta, GA: Centers for Disease Control and Prevention (US); 2011 [updated 2013 April 17]. Available at: www.cdc.gov/socialmedia/tools/guidelines/index.html (accessed 29 October 2013).
32. Innes E. *The Rise of Dr Google: half of Britons now get health advice online rather than seeing their GP.* Mail Online; 2013 Mar 20 [updated 2013 Mar 21]. Available at: www.dailymail.

co.uk/health/article-2296398/The-rise-Dr-Google-Half-Britons-health-advice-online-seeing-GP.html (accessed 29 October 2013).

33. Pew Internet & American Life Project (US). *Health Online 2013*. Washington, DC: Pew Research Center (US); 2013 [updated 2013 Jan 15]. Available at: www.pewinternet.org/Reports/2013/Health-online.aspx (accessed 29 October 2013).

34. Pew Internet & American Life Project (US). *Mobile Health 2012*. Washington, DC: Pew Research Center (US); 2012 [updated 2012 Nov 8]. Available at: www.pewinternet.org/Reports/2012/Mobile-Health.aspx (accessed 29 October 2013).

35. PriceWaterhouseCoopers (US). *Social Media 'Likes' Healthcare: from marketing to social business*. New York, NY: PriceWaterhouseCoopers LLC (US); 2012. Available at: www.pwc.com/us/en/health-industries/publications/health-care-social-media.jhtml (accessed 29 October 2013).

36. Gudnadottir U, Fritz J, Zerbel S, *et al*. Reducing health care-associated infections: patients want to be engaged and learn about infection prevention. *Am J Infect Control*. 2013; **41**(11): 955–8.

37. McGuckin M, Govednik J, Hyman D, *et al*. Public reporting of health care-associated infection rates: are consumers aware and engaged? *Infect Control Hosp Epidemiol*. 2013; **34**(11): 1201–3.

38. McDonald KM, Chang C, Schultz E. *Through the Quality Kaleidoscope: reflections on the science and practice of improving health care quality. Closing the quality gap: revisiting the state of the science. Methods Research Report*. AHRQ Publication No. 13-EHC041-EF. Rockville, MD: Agency for Healthcare Research and Quality; 2013.

CHAPTER 16

The role of healthcare culture in patient safety

Dave Grewcock, Aidan Halligan and Yogi Amin

There is often something close to outrage in the political and media debates that surround high-profile safety failures in the National Health Service (NHS) – a sense of disbelief that nationally regulated, publicly funded, twenty-first-century organisations can apparently fail to apply even the most basic safety checks to those in their care. How can a hospital staffed by compassionate, highly educated individuals manage to execute an audacious surgical procedure, only for the patient to succumb to a deep vein thrombosis for want of some routine observations and a pair of compression stockings? How is it that a clinical team can invest so much effort in stabilising a frail, elderly man after a fall, and then send him to a ward that seemingly fails to ensure he has enough to drink? Why do patients succumb to infections when in many cases all that is needed is some low-cost handwash and good hand hygiene practice?

In a broad sense, we now understand much more about how failure originates in and propagates through complex systems.[1] In some instances this understanding has driven the innovation of new medical devices that 'design out' the risk of failure. The practice of adopting 'designed incompatibility' can now make it impossible, for example, to connect an air pump to a patient's intravenous line. However, such examples remain inevitably in the minority. Most healthcare processes are more critically dependent on components that cannot be fundamentally redesigned: human beings.

Thanks largely to progress in other domains, particularly aviation, we now understand much more about the 'human factors' that constrain our individual performance – our cognitive biases, the limits on our memory and attention, the effects of tiredness and distraction, the ambiguity inherent in our communication[2] – but even that leaves us well short of a comprehensive description of what determines patient safety. To a large degree, patient safety is a function of the attitude, judgements, beliefs and behaviour of healthcare staff because, ultimately, it is these factors that determine whether policy and procedure are adhered to, whether professional standards of practice are applied, and whether shortcomings in care become tolerated as 'unavoidable' or 'insignificant'. How an individual behaves is, of course, contingent not just on his or her own particular beliefs or cognitive characteristics, but also on the beliefs, attitudes and behaviours of those around the individual. From this subtle, shifting complex of interactions between the individual and the group emerges a set of shared but unwritten – and often unconscious and usually unspoken – set of behavioural standards that shape how work is done and, in healthcare, how patients are treated and cared for. This is 'organisational' or 'workplace culture', and over the last 2 decades it has come to be understood both as the most intractable limit on the quality and safety of care and as the richest source of potential improvement.[3]

Most of the reports into serious healthcare care failure in the last 20 years – Bristol Royal Infirmary[4] and Mid Staffordshire NHS Foundation Trust[5,6] being seminal examples – have identified some element of 'poor' or 'dysfunctional' organisational culture as a significant contributory factor, and the creation of a 'good' culture is the imperative behind much of what is written about good leadership.[7]

Most healthcare staff will now readily acknowledge that 'workplace culture' is a critical determinant of how safe our patients are – even if they cannot describe with any great rigor or precision what culture is, the mechanism of its impact on safety, or how culture can be changed. Although formal definitions of culture exist – the Francis report refer to 'the predominating attitudes and behaviour that characterise the functioning of a group or organisation'[5] – most of us have become comfortable with the informal shorthand that culture is 'the way things are done around here'; not least because it often resonates with our own personal experience. We have all witnessed teams being endlessly and silently creative in subverting or undermining change initiatives that they perceive as 'unacceptable'. For those concerned with maintaining or enhancing patient safety – and in fact any change programme – the conclusions are obvious, and a little sobering: to ignore the cultural dimension of our efforts is fundamentally to jeopardise them.

Yet the cultural aspects of safety and quality improvement are routinely disregarded, even by senior, experienced leaders. In our own NHS careers, we have witnessed a number of safety- and quality-related initiatives launched and brought, sadly, to compromised or incomplete conclusion, all without any considered effort to address, or even assess, the cultural dimension to the change. There are a variety of reasons.

Some managers and leaders hold fast to the view that although culture and its impact are significant and real, it is nonetheless not a legitimate topic for 'real work'. For them, culture is too nebulous a concept to engage with directly, or even describe. They would hold that culture is an entirely emergent property; it arises from a particular place and group and can be tolerated or accommodated but, except at the extremes, cannot essentially be changed.

Others argue that culture can indeed be shaped, at least approximately, and that a set of familiar managerial interventions is sufficient for the purpose. Often this translates to a belief that merely describing the desired culture – for instance, in the form of a 'values' or 'mission' statement – will be enough to bring that culture into being. Or they believe that it can be 'instructed' into existence through a set of policies and procedures that determine how individuals and groups should behave. For this constituency of thought, shaping workplace culture is a matter of reviewing and refining policies, issuing information and instructions, and closer management.

However, for most the disinclination to address cultural issues has a much simpler explanation: they seem overwhelmingly, impossibly complex to tackle. If culture is that set of collective attitudes and behaviours that emerge from all the actions and interactions of an often heterogeneous group of individuals, then surely the dynamics of 'cultural intervention' are simply too complex to compute? Better, then, to set aside culture as a given, focus on those things we feel we can change more predictably – money, resource, system design – and satisfy ourselves that we have done the best we can in the circumstances of a complex world.

While they are understandable, such conclusions encourage leaders to discount and disregard issues of culture too frequently, and thereby to tolerate and legitimise lower standards of safety and quality than might otherwise be achieved: our view is that these conclusions need to be challenged.

The phenomenon of culture is not so nebulous that it cannot be described. In our own work we return repeatedly to the concept of the 'high reliability organisation',[8] an idea that is familiar to some in healthcare but which has yet to fully penetrate the thinking of health service leaders.[9] While not a complete description of an 'ideal' healthcare culture – it says nothing about the qualities of compassion and kindness that most of us would wish to see – it does describe the attributes of cultures that assure demonstrably high levels of safety in complex, safety-critical domains – aircraft carrier operation, air traffic control and nuclear power generation being examples. The 'high reliability organisation' model describes, for instance, how safety-critical cultures foster a 'preoccupation with failure' – an intense focus on why and how individual failures occur and what can be learned from them. The form of this 'preoccupation' is more than simply the creation of processes to capture, record and analyse failure; it is a cultural 'stance', an automatic, reflexive and dispassionate interest in the diagnostic value of failure. Sometimes, the contrast with the cultural attitude to failure in healthcare could hardly be more distinct. For all the formal incident reporting systems that exist in healthcare, except in the most serious instances the common cultural response is not to scrutinise failure, but simply to survive it, compensate and carry on. The contrast is instructive, but our real purpose for now is simply to help dispel the misconception that culture is too nebulous to engage with: cultures do contrast between sectors and organisations and can be described with some rigor.

The second misconception, that culture can be 'engineered' into being through the right set of systems and policies, is harder to deconstruct and proves seductive to many of those charged with improving safety. The near iconic infection control work of Peter Pronovost and his collaborators,[10] provides ample example. Convinced that intravenous catheter-related infections in his intensive care unit could be cut, Pronovost began to research best practice in line insertion and management, and compared it both with his own practice and that of colleagues. He settled on five evidence-based practices – simple measures such as properly draping the patient and using the most effective hand-cleaning products before the procedure – that significantly reduced the risk of line infection. At that point, on average, only 30% of line insertions on his unit adhered to all five of these measures; there were issues with the supply of hand sanitiser, the location of equipment, and the individual understanding and behaviour of some of his colleagues. Pronovost and his colleagues designed an intervention to improve adherence to good practice. Equipment trolleys were relocated and properly organised, senior executives were lobbied to ensure that the organisation bought the right hand hygiene products, and short educational sessions were run to ensure staff understood the significance of the measures. The five practices were assembled into a checklist, and nursing staff were asked to ensure that their medical colleagues applied the checklist for all non-emergency line insertions. The results were astonishing by any measure. In the space of 3 months, the catheter-associated infection rate fell to near zero and although it later rose slightly, it was undeniable that Pronovost's intervention had had a sustained impact. It was reckoned that some 1500 lives and $200 million in healthcare costs were saved in the state of Michigan during the first 18 months of the project. Understandably, the programme generated huge excitement and, ultimately, was successfully transplanted into other organisations in the same state, across the United States, and beyond. However, the transplant was never straight-forward. In trying to replicate his work, other teams adopted the mechanics of his intervention, but not always its ethos. New collaborators focused on the tangibles of the programme – the principles of equipment organisation, the type of hand sanitisers and, above all, the checklist of measures. In fact, as part of his programme, Pronovost and his team had been engaged in a sophisticated and often challenging programme of cultural change. Medical peers who were reluctant to implement his changes were engaged in robust debate. The nursing staff who had been asked to challenge the practice of senior medical staff when they were failing, for instance, to use the checklist, inevitably found themselves set against established cultural norms about the relative authority of nursing and medical staff. The nurses were given senior executive support, and instructions to bleep Pronovost personally if his fellow medics were unwilling to comply. These aspects of the intervention seemed less palatable to those organisations seeking to adopt Pronovost's programme.

These new, but selective, adopters had chosen to discount or recoil from the cultural aspects of the programme and gravitated instead toward the apparatus of change – checklists, educational programmes, better systems of organisation, and so forth. There was nothing wrong with that apparatus and, indeed, part of Pronovost's intervention was a staff programme on the 'science of safety' that dealt with the theoretical basis of safety and change. However, fundamentally, new adopters were succumbing to the notion that their organisations were machines that could best be steered by the right combination of managerial inputs. This view owes much to the nineteenth- or twentieth-century image of the organisation such as a factory or production line, where, historically, relatively simple shifts in input, time, resource and manpower could have a predictable, linear effect on 'output'. Always a simplifi-cation, this image holds even less well for modern knowledge-based organisations, especially healthcare organisations, but it nonetheless has a tenacious hold on our imaginations.

The organisational 'response' of modern enterprise is more contingent on the choices made by its individual staff. The levers of command and control now have rather narrow, easily exceeded limits. We are, more than ever, expected to decide individually or locally what work needs doing, how it should be done and how we invest our energies. These choices are obviously influenced by our own personal values and principals, and by the loyalties we hold. They can be distorted by the mistaken assumptions we make and by similar 'self-imposed' limits.

This is particularly and profoundly true of healthcare organisations, populated as they are by independently minded, sophisticated thinkers, at least originally motivated by a deep sense of personal vocation, and schooled in professions that have strong histories and traditions. Our healthcare organisations are actually often complex mosaics of subcultures, each one a reflection of a particular group of staff, their local personalities and leaders, and the immediately local history of their service. Not surprisingly, then, the cultural response to a given intervention can be led or guided, but rarely steered by instruction 'from above'.

However, we also dissent from the view that 'healthcare culture' – because it cannot simply be mandated into a particular shape – is simply too complex and unpredictable to be worth engaging with. Our own contribution to the infection control effort is to advocate for the routine use of a checklist during hospital inpatient rounds and perhaps other key clinical processes such as shift handover and team briefings.[11] The 'ward safety' checklist is not dissimilar to the Pronovost initiative or the World Health Organization safer surgery checklist[12]: it aims to encourage greater uniformity in the checking of known inpatient risk factors – does the patient have the correct deep vein thrombosis prophylaxis, have fluid balance and drug charts been checked, is the patient at risk of falls, and so on? There are a number of infection control-related items on the list – meticillin-resistant *Staphylococcus aureus* status, infection risk and antibiotic control, for instance – but we cite it here not so much as a solution to infection control, but rather as an example of an alternative view of culture and culture change. The checklist provides a succinct summary of routine, daily inpatient checks, and, if no other preference exists, an entirely serviceable template for the structure of a ward round. However, the ward round is a complex process, having to accommodate an enormous range of circumstances, disciplines and patient needs, and the checklist is not a prescription. To rigidly dictate a particular style and approach to the checklist would be to cut too crudely across the autonomy of the individuals and teams involved. It would risk disrupting the custom and practices of teams that already deliver safe and effective rounds, and it would discount and ignore some of the difficult constraints under which staff work. Edicts would at best encourage superficial compliance, and at worst outright and irreversible rejection by the staff involved, perhaps resulting in a net loss rather than a gain in patient safety. So while the checklist offers a style and structure for rounds, it does not mandate one: there are no signature spaces, and no boxes to check. Instead, teams are encouraged to discover their own best implementation of the checklist.

The checklist is simply a token, a prompt for individuals and teams to begin to assess issues of attitude to risk, variation in practice, human factors, communication and professional dynamics. It is about helping staff to appreciate that safety is improved through systematic attention to the basic, often unglamorous aspects of, in this case, inpatient care. Ultimately, the aim is to challenge staff to assess and perhaps revise their individual and shared assumptions about why the 'system' is preventing them from delivering the standard of care they instinctively feel is achievable.

For us, the ward safety checklist is not merely a checklist but, rather, a culture change effort, one that departs from the common assumptions about culture change that we have described here, and it is fundamentally more optimistic. It is predicated on the belief that healthcare culture change enjoys one critical advantage when compared with other domains: the very deep values base of its staff. Only a small minority of the failures in healthcare stem from casual negligence, lack of care, or bad intent; for the most part, healthcare staff have an instinctive sense of what should be done to protect their patient, and a genuine desire to deliver the best care possible. What perturbs them from that course are the perceived constraints that our healthcare organisations appear to place on their actions – constraints that often transpire to be self-imposed and which are often learned, mistakenly, as the key to professional and career survival.

We would do nothing to suggest that culture change is anything but difficult. The shared pattern of assumptions, beliefs and behaviours can, indeed, be incredibly complex, and reshaping them is beyond any simple process engineering. However, healthcare culture can be changed. It is a matter of understanding the natural attractors that shape individual decisions and guiding individuals and groups back to their natural, originally motivated instincts. It may involve some organisational engineering to remove overt barriers, but more often than not it means designing an environment – which may be something as simple as, in our case, a checklist – that cues and facilitates the behaviour that healthcare staff want, instinctively, to engage in.

It is with great regret that we share with you the loss of Aiden who sadly passed away before the publication of this book. There is no doubt that Aiden will be very much missed and that the preceding chapter will form one very small part of the monumental contribution he made to the field of safety and quality both nationally and internationally.

REFERENCES

1. Reason J. *Managing the Risks of Organizational Accidents*. London: Ashgate; 1997.
2. Carthey J, Clarke J. *Implementing Human Factors in Healthcare: 'how to' guide*. London: Patient Safety First Campaign; 2010. Available at: www.patientsafetyfirst.nhs.uk/ashx/Asset. ashx?path=/Intervention-support/Human+Factors+How-to+Guide+v1.2.pdf (accessed 4 June 2015).

3. Halligan A. Patient safety: culture eats strategy for breakfast. *Br J Hosp Med (Lond).* 2011; **72**(10): 548–9.

4. Kennedy I. *Learning from Bristol: public inquiry into children's heart surgery at the Bristol Royal Infirmary 1984–1995.* CM 5207. London: The Stationery Office; 2001.

5. Francis R. *Independent Inquiry into Care Provided by Mid Staffordshire NHS Foundation Trust January 2005–March 2009.* London: The Stationery Office; 2010.

6. Francis R. *Report of the Mid Staffordshire NHS Foundation Trust Public Inquiry.* London: The Stationery Office; 2013.

7. Halligan A. The need for an NHS staff college. *J R Soc Med.* 2010; **103**(10): 387–91.

8. Weick KE, Sutcliffe KM. *Managing the Unexpected: resilient performance in an age of uncertainty.* 2nd ed. San Francisco, CA: Jossey-Bass; 2007.

9. The Health Foundation. *High Reliability Organisations.* London: The Health Foundation; 2011. Available at: www.health.org.uk/public/cms/75/76/313/3070/High%20reliability%20 organisations.pdf?realName=PngyC6.pdf (accessed 4 June 2015)

10. Pronovost P, Vohr E. *Safe Patients, Smart Hospitals: how one doctor's checklist can help us change healthcare from the inside out.* New York, NY: Plume Books; 2010.

11. Amin Y, Grewcock D, Andrews S, *et al.* Why patients need leaders: introducing a ward safety checklist. *J R Soc Med.* 2012; **105**(9): 377–83.

12. Haynes AB, Weiser TG, Berry WR, *et al.* A surgical safety checklist to reduce morbidity and mortality in a global population. *N Engl J Med.* 2009; **360**(5): 491–9.

CHAPTER 17

Is outcome surveillance of healthcare-associated infections really necessary?

. . . .

Nizam Damani

The word 'surveillance' comes from a French phrase meaning 'watching over'.[1] The word surveillance has negative connotations, as nobody likes to be *watched over*, either as an individual or as a group. Surveillance is an essential component of the infection prevention and control (IPC) programme, as its main aim is to reduce the risk of patients getting healthcare-associated infections (HCAIs).[2] Surveillance of HCAIs can be performed by counting infections (*outcome surveillance*) and/or monitoring processes (*process surveillance*) (*see* Figure 17.1).

It has been estimated that about 5%–10% of patients admitted to modern hospitals in the developed world acquire one or more HCAIs; the proportion can exceed 25% in low- to middle-income countries. The risk of acquiring HCAIs in developing countries is 2–20 times higher than in developed countries.[3] It has been estimated that if good IPC practices are applied, more than 70% of HCAIs are preventable.[4-6]

LIMITATIONS AND PITFALLS OF OUTCOME SURVEILLANCE
Active versus passive surveillance

A surveillance process can be *active*, with a process for seeking out HCAI cases, or it can be *passive*, which is dependent on a third party to fill out a form or chart and send it in to the IPC team for analysis. Reliance on passive surveillance has been clearly demonstrated to underestimate cases.[8] However, active surveillance requires

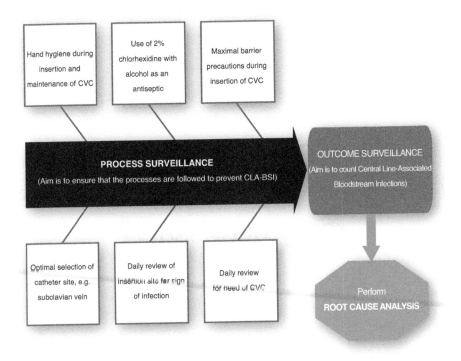

FIGURE 17.1 The difference between process and outcome surveillance (adapted, with modifications, from Damani[7])

CVC, central venous catheter; CLA-BSI, central line-associated bloodstream infection

a substantial amount of time and, consequently, fewer resources are directed toward the implementation of good IPC practices to prevent HCAIs in the first place!

Reliance on good-quality laboratory service

The implementation of outcome surveillance requires the support of a good-quality laboratory service, which can be a major issue, especially in low- to middle-income countries.[2,9] In addition, most definitions of HCAIs require standardised methods of processing of microbiology specimens and, because of a lack of internationally agreed methodology, this may not always be achievable.

Problem with definitions

There are *no internationally agreed definitions* on outcome surveillance, and various countries have developed their own definitions and surveillance systems. The definitions developed by the Centers for Disease Control and Prevention (CDC)/

National Healthcare Safety Network[10] and the European Centre for Disease Prevention and Control[11] have been most commonly used in the United States and Europe, respectively. In addition, there is also a discrepancy between the *epidemiological* and the *clinical diagnosis* of HCAIs. Recently, a prospective study compared CDC ventilator-associated pneumonia (VAP) infection rates with VAP infection rates calculated using the American College of Chest Physicians' definition of VAP. The study involved 2060 ventilated patients; 12 cases of VAP were identified using CDC criteria, whereas 83 cases were identified using the American College of Chest Physicians' criteria – that is, 1.2 versus 8.5 cases per 1000 ventilator days, respectively.[12]

It is well recognised that the application of HCAI *definitions is complex* and requires subjective judgement for interpretation – the correct application for the diagnosis of VAP is notoriously difficult and it is recommended that the measurement of processes should be used to reduce VAP.[13] Therefore, it is essential that the personnel who are responsible for collection of data require *substantive training* and *practice* to develop proficiency to help reduce subjectivity and promote consistency. A recent study has highlighted the need for an *independent validation* of outcome data, as it observed that CDC / National Healthcare Safety Network central line–associated bloodstream infection (CLA-BSI) surveillance definitions are prone to misinterpretation, and it reported overall sensitivity of hospital reporting of CLA-BSIs as 72%.[14]

Although *automated surveillance* is more cost-effective and may provide more consistent information, its applicability depends on the way in which healthcare is provided in a particular region or country, making comparison even more difficult.[15]

Risk stratification of data

Since the patient populations and procedures vary substantially from hospital to hospital,[15] it is essential that HCAI rates are risk-adjusted for the most important known confounding factors, as reporting crude data will not explain variations between various healthcare facilities and it is essential for public reporting of HCAIs. It is important to note that the current methods of risk-adjustment for various patient categories represent a compromise and do not account for all known potential confounding variables. In addition, collecting data is very time-consuming, because data must be collected on the *entire* population at risk (the denominator), rather than on only the fraction with a HCAI (the numerator); therefore, it can be argued that if the number of HCAIs in a unit is low, risk adjustment may not be worthwhile.[16]

Follow-up of patients

Current medical advances and change in the delivery of healthcare have allowed shorter stays in hospital with higher throughput of patients.[17] Therefore, most HCAIs will not be identified during the hospital stay and will appear *after* the patient has been discharged. It has been estimated that between 14% and 70% of surgical site infections (SSIs) occur after discharge.[17] Therefore, post-discharge surveillance of all HCAIs is essential to obtain accurate data; however, the best way to conduct post-discharge surveillance in a manner that is both efficient and cost-effective remains a matter of debate and is rarely performed, even in high-resource countries where surveillance programmes have been well established for decades.

Does feedback of data on outcome surveillance *really* reduce HCAI rates?

Published data in the literature cite examples where feedback of outcome surveillance to the clinical team has resulted in a reduction of HCAI rates, but these reductions are modest and the exact reasons for these reductions have not been rigorously studied. The most reliable study cited in the literature on the impact of reduction of SSIs was led by Professor Peter Cruse, a professor of surgery.[18] It is important to note that this study was not led by an epidemiologist or an infection control practitioner. After conducting outcome surveillance, his team analysed the data and spearheaded changes in surgical practice (*process change*), which led to a substantial reduction of SSIs. Currently, in almost all countries, the individuals who collect the outcome surveillance data worldwide have neither full understanding and/or knowledge of the processes *nor* any influence to change the clinical practice.

It is well recognised that the reporting of surveillance data can increase awareness and this pressure to 'look good' could motivate hospitals to *under-report* HCAI rates. For example, there is evidence that some of the reduction in CLA-BSI rates is due to *reinterpretations* of surveillance definitions in the post-surveillance period.[19] In addition, the US players such as the Centers for Medicare and Medicaid Services increasingly use patient safety indicators to reward hospitals with lower complication rates in pay for performance initiatives, and introduction of these measures may introduce bias with temptation to under-report HCAIs. Furthermore, publications in literature are biased toward success stories, often missing possibly more frequent failures due to lack of submission or rejection.[20]

TABLE 17.1 Process versus outcome surveillance: summary of advantages[2,5–7,15–17]

	Process surveillance	Outcome surveillance
Objective	Prevent infection by implementing and monitoring good IPC practices	Count infections by applying agreed definitions for HCAIs
Need support of good-quality microbiology laboratory to diagnose HCAIs	No	Yes
Education and training	Yes	Yes
	Education and training is required to implement and monitor standardised IPC practices	Education and training is required to interpret and apply definition consistently
Help embed good IPC practices in the unit or hospital	Yes	No
Immediately identify break in good IPC practices	Yes	No
Clinical judgement	No clinical judgement is required, as compliance is monitored against best IPC practices (e.g. by using checklist or HCAI care bundles)	Clinical judgement is required subject to interpretation of case definitions of HCAIs
Risk adjustment of data is required	No	Yes
Data are affected by patient characteristics, case ascertainment, definitions and risk factors	No	Yes
Application of statistical test is necessary because HCAI rates are subject to random variation and are influenced by number of cases and frequency with which outcome occurs	No	Yes
Rate affected by early discharge of patients	No	Yes
Measurement of data	More sensitive	Less sensitive

(*continued*)

	Process surveillance	Outcome surveillance
Data is relatively easier and less costly to collect and interpret	Yes	No
Aspects of care	Aspects of care quality are measured by implementation of good IPC practice on *all* patients	Aspects of care are measured by rate of HCAIs in selected patients

IPC, infection control and prevention; HCAI, healthcare-associated infections

Table 17.1 summarises the advantages of process *versus* outcome surveillance. In addition, effective implementation of process surveillance has the following added advantages.

- Monitoring compliance is more effective, as 'people do what you inspect, not necessarily what you expect.'[29]
- The introduction of standardised protocols, procedures and good IPC practices help avoid variation in practices caused by high turnover of clinical staff in the unit and/or hospital.
- Process monitoring allows the clinical team to understand, learn and implement good practices that not only serve as an educational tool but also are applied to *every* eligible patient.
- Lapses and breach in the protocol are recognised and addressed more quickly before an increase in the infection rate has occurred.
- Failure in process measurement focuses on the analysis and investigation of the individual infection rather than seeking to interpret statistical variations in HCAI rates.

ADVANTAGES AND LIMITATIONS OF PROCESS SURVEILLANCE

Although industry has shown us for decades that *reducing process variation* directly *influences the final product defect rate*,[21-23] it was only a few years ago that this concept was translated into clinical practice. This was undertaken through the introduction of the care bundle by the US Institute for Healthcare Improvement,[24] later modified and adopted by the UK Department of Health.[25] A care bundle is described as 'a grouping of best practices with respect to a disease process that individually improves care, but when applied together results in substantially greater improvements.'[24]

It is recommended that compliance with all the elements of the care bundle should be measured on an 'all or nothing' basis.[26] This is because the temptation to pick only easier elements of the care bundle is too great. Although compliance with all elements of the HCAI care bundle on all patients at all times is ideal, it can be very difficult to achieve in practice. It has been highlighted that if an average intensive care unit were to comply with at least one component of the care bundle at all times, they would experience an estimated 38% decrease in their CLA-BSI rate.[19]

It is recognised that implementation of HCAI care bundles has its limitations and they have not been subjected to rigorous scientific scrutiny in published medical literature. However, their introduction has led to a paradigm shift in IPC practices, as more emphasis is now being placed on embedding good IPC practices, harnessing support from senior managers, and addressing and overcoming barriers among the clinician team to achieve a substantial and sustained reduction in HCAIs.[5,6,26–28]

However, effective implementation of good practice has its own challenges, and the question today is not 'what to do?' but rather, 'how to do it?'[5] Experience has shown that the clinical team might develop a 'tick the box' mentality to filling in the checklist. However, this issue can be overcome by monitoring and analysing the reliability of surveillance data to show a reduction in HCAIs, and if this is not achieved then it will help to open up discussion with the relevant clinical team and help them understand the issues and barriers to implementation. Once the units have successfully achieved these objectives, then only numerator data can be collected for outcome surveillance and *all preventable* HCAIs should be subjected to root cause analysis (RCA).

ROOT CAUSE ANALYSIS

RCA is based on the concept that adverse events are minimised and/or eliminated by identifying the real issue and taking corrective action to eliminate the *root causes* rather than merely addressing the immediately obvious issues that have resulted in HCAIs. RCA has been successfully applied in the United Kingdom to reduce and sustain reduction in both meticillin-resistant *Staphylococcus aureus* bacteraemia and *Clostridium difficile* infections.* The Root Cause Analysis Toolkit and eLearning Programme is available from the UK National Patient Safety Agency website.†

The most common way to perform RCA is to use the '5 Whys' technique, whereby the person asks a question five times to explore the cause and effect, to determine the *root cause* of the problem. Since the failure does not always occur in a linear pattern and, more often, multiple factors combine in parallel, a fishbone

---

* www.gov.uk/government/organisations/public-health-england
† http://npsa.nhs.uk

diagram – where the spine of the fish represents the sequence of events leading to an adverse outcome – can be used. For successful RCA, it is essential that the analysis is carried out by a clinical team and assertion must be backed up by the evidence. Information gathered by the RCA over a long period may make it useful as a *proactive method* and, if effectively carried out, it can be used as tool for *continuous improvement* to reduce HCAIs.

CONCLUSION

In conclusion, unlike other industries, the approach adopted by the healthcare institution worldwide historically relied more on measuring outcome only (HCAI rates), creating benchmarks and national averages, and proudly publishing league tables comparing various hospitals. This approach has resulted in an acceptance among clinicians that, among other complications, getting HCAIs is a part of modern healthcare delivery. However, informing a patient that your hospital has a lower rate of HCAIs than the national average or benchmark is not satisfactory from the patient's perspective, as when a patient gets a HCAI, the rate for that given patient is 100%!

The primary objective of surveillance is to assist in reducing the risk of preventable HCAIs, and for surveillance to be effective it is essential that the IPC programme must not rely on outcome surveillance alone. Gathering data on the outcome indicators is complicated, cumbersome, prone to subjective interpretation, and does not provide information on the proportion of preventable infections, or provide guidance on what action must be taken to prevent HCAIs in the first place. For a substantial and sustained reduction of HCAI rates, it is essential for us to place greater emphasis on implementing and monitoring good IPC practices (process surveillance) and performing RCA on *all preventable* HCAIs while maintaining successful traditional features of outcome surveillance. Hospitals which have successfully implemented and embedded good IPC practice are now counting 'infection free' days since the last HCAI, instead of benchmarking their traditional HCAI rates using outcome surveillance.

REFERENCES

1. Wikipedia. *Surveillance.* http://en.wikipedia.org/wiki/Surveillance (accessed 7 September 2012).
2. Damani N. Surveillance of health care associated infections in low to middle resource countries. *Int J Infect Control.* 2012; **8**: i4.

3. World Health Organization (WHO). *Report on the Burden of Endemic Health Care-Associated Infection Worldwide.* Geneva: WHO; 2011.

4. Umscheid CA, Mitchell MD, Doshi JA, *et al.* Estimating the proportion of healthcare-associated infections that are reasonably preventable and the related mortality and costs. *Infect Control Hosp Epidemiol.* 2011; **32**(2): 101–14.

5. Zingg W, Walder B, Pittet D. Prevention of catheter-related infection: toward zero risk? *Curr Opin Infect Dis.* 2011; **24**(4): 377–84.

6. Klompas M. Is a ventilator-associated pneumonia rate of zero really possible? *Curr Opin Infect Dis.* 2012; **25**(2): 176–82.

7. Damani NN. *Manual of Infection Prevention and Control.* 3rd ed. Oxford: Oxford University Press; 2012.

8. Scheckler WE. Surveillance, foundation for the future: a historical overview and evolution of methodologies. *Am J Infect Control.* 1997; **25**(2): 106–11.

9. Damani NN. Surveillance in countries with limited resources. *Int J Infect Control.* 2008; **4**: 1.

10. Horan TC, Andrus M, Margaret A. CDC/NHSN surveillance definition of health care-associated infection and criteria for specific types of infections in the acute care setting. *Am J Infect Control.* 2008; **36**(5): 309–32.

11. Hospitals in Europe Link for Infection Control through Surveillance (HELICS). *Surveillance of Nosocomial Infections in Intensive Care Units.* HELICS; 2004. Available at: http://ecdc.europa.eu/en/activities/surveillance/HAI/Documents/0409_IPSE_ICU_protocol.pdf (accessed 7 September 2012).

12. Skrupky LP, McConnell K, Dallas J, *et al.* A comparison of ventilator associated pneumonia rates as identified according to the National Healthcare Safety Network and American College of Chest Physicians criteria. *Crit Care Med.* 2012; **40**(1): 281–4.

13. Klompas M, Platt R. Ventilator-associated pneumonia – the wrong quality measure for benchmarking. *Ann Intern Med.* 2007; **147**(11): 803–5.

14. Oh JY, Cunningham MC, Beldavs ZG, *et al.* Statewide validation of hospital-reported central line-associated bloodstream infections: Oregon, 2009. *Infect Control Hosp Epidemiol.* 2012; **33**(5): 439–45.

15. O'Neill E, Humphreys H. Use of surveillance data for prevention of healthcare-associated infection: risk adjustment and reporting dilemmas. *Curr Opin Infect Dis.* 2009; **22**(4): 359–63.

16. Tokars JI, Richards C, Andrus M, *et al.* The changing face of surveillance for health care-associated infections. *Clin Infect Dis.* 2004; **39**(9): 1347–52.

17. Delgado-Rodriguez M, Gomez-Ortega A, Sillero-Arenas M, *et al.* Epidemiology of surgical-site infections diagnosed after hospital discharge: a prospective cohort study. *Infect Control Hosp Epidemiol.* 2001; **22**(1): 24–30.

18. Cruse PJ, Foord R. The epidemiology of wound infection: a 10-year prospective study of 62,939 wounds. *Surg Clin North Am.* 1980; **60**(1): 27–40.

19. Furya EY, Dick A, Perencevich EN, *et al.* Central line bundle implementation in the US ICUs and impact of blood stream infection. *PLoS.* 2011; **6**(1): e15452.

20. Goldacre B. *Bad Science.* London: Fourth Estate; 2008.

21. Walton M. *The Deming Management Method.* New York, NY: Putnam Publishing; 1986.

22. Crosby PB. *Quality without Tears: the art of hassle-free management.* New York, NY: McGraw-Hill; 1984.

23. Mant J. Process versus outcome indicators in assessment of quality of health care. *Int J Qual Health Care.* 2001; **3**(6): 475–80.

24. Institute for Healthcare Improvement. *Infection Prevention Bundles*. Available at: www.ihi. org/topics/bundles/Pages/default.aspx (accessed 7 September 2012).

25. UK Department of Health. *Using High Impact Interventions: using care bundles to reduce healthcare associated infection by increasing reliability and safety.* London: Department of Health; 2007.

26. Berenholtz SM, Pronovost PJ, Lipsett PA, *et al.* Eliminating catheter-related bloodstream infections in the intensive care unit. *Crit Care Med.* 2004; **32**(10): 2014–20.

27. Pronovost P, Needham D, Berenholtz S, *et al.* An intervention to decrease catheter-related bloodstream infections in the ICU. *N Engl J Med.* 2006; **355**(26): 2725–32.

28. Pronovost PJ, Goeschel CA, Colantuoni E, *et al.* Sustaining reductions in catheter related bloodstream infections in Michigan intensive care units: observational study. *BMJ.* 2010; **340**: c309.

29. Crow S. Methods of surveillance and presentation of data. In: Gurevich I, Tafuro P, Chuha BA, editors. *The Theory and Practice of Infection Control.* New York: Praeger; 1984. pp. 15–27.

Conclusion

Within this book we have tried to bring to the forefront a range of differing perceptions and perspectives that are diverse, challenging and thought-provoking. Our intention has been to present infection prevention and control as an overarching process, one that goes beyond the simplistic standpoint of it just being about hand hygiene. Rather, infection prevention and control is a process that affects us all in many ways with regard to each individual's right to health, wellbeing and life. In reading through the differing chapters of this book, we hope you will have started to realise that infection prevention and control is a multifaceted and highly complex combination of physical, psychological, social, socioeconomic and political processes internationally. No one person, group, organisation or country can consider itself to exist in isolation where IP&C is concerned. IP&C is a global issue and, for that matter, problem. Further, infection prevention and control is not something that can simply be paid lip service; it is not an incidental to be enacted at the convenience of individuals, management or organisations after something has gone wrong or, for example, when a visit from an external authority is expected. Infection prevention and control must always be proactive and preventive in nature, as opposed to a retroactive and curative set of actions and reactions.

Index

CPD with Radcliffe

You can now use a selection of our books to achieve CPD (Continuing Professional Development) points through directed reading.

We provide a free online form and downloadable certificate for your appraisal portfolio. Look for the CPD logo and register with us at: www.radcliffehealth.com/cpd

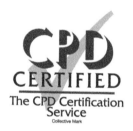

Printed and bound by CPI Group (UK) Ltd, Croydon, CR0 4YY

23/10/2024

01777678-0006